"In countries where complex and sometimes confusing nursing theories are taught, this book will help Christian nurses see the forest *and* the trees. It may also help non-Christian nurses understand how and why Christians function in the way they do. I have nurses in several countries on my mental list of people to whom I will send a copy."

PAT ASHWORTH, M.Sc., R.G.N., R.M., FRCN,
former senior lecturer in nursing, University of Ulster, Northern Ireland;
former president, Nurses Christian Fellowship International

"Dr. Shelly and Dr. Miller have interwoven church history, the history of nursing, views of selected nurse theorists, views of various religions, and theological concepts of Christianity to present a Christian worldview for nursing. Through the use of stories they illustrate what nursing practice can be when it is based on this worldview. It is a useful guidebook for nursing students, graduate nurses and caregivers from other health care professions."

EDNA M. FORDYCE, Ed.D., R.N., C.S.-P,
professor emeritus, department of nursing, Towson State University

"This book beautifully fills a critical void in the professional literature related to the philosophy of nursing. Shelly and Miller have taken the core and calling of nursing—*caring*—and clearly shown that this calling is in jeopardy unless motivated by Christian commitment. Their many clinical examples show how a perspective founded on biblical principles is applicable to any and all nursing situations."

PHYLLIS S. KARNS, R.N., Ph.D.,
dean, Baylor University School of Nursing

"A marvelous integration of theological commitment and nursing practice, this book is just what a Christian theology of nursing should be. The authors argue so effectively that nursing at its best—recognized as a vocation, or calling, of God— is not just any sort of caring but caring with a God-directed content and character."

JOHN F. KILNER, Ph.D.,
director, The Center for Bioethics and Human Dignity

"This book is inspired. The biblical worldview of a personal God is central to the entire text. It offers *shalom;* it offers the hope of Jesus Christ. It is a healing experience to read this book."

ELIZABETH STERNDALE, president, ASDAN-NAD
(formerly Association of Seventh-day Adventist Nurses)

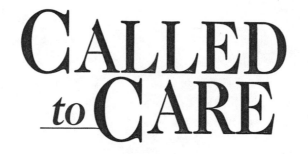

CALLED to CARE

A Christian Theology of Nursing

JUDITH ALLEN SHELLY
& ARLENE B. MILLER

InterVarsity Press
Downers Grove, Illinois

InterVarsity Press
P.O. Box 1400, Downers Grove, IL 60515
World Wide Web: www.ivpress.com
E-mail: mail@ivpress.com

InterVarsity Press® is the book-publishing division of InterVarsity Christian Fellowship/USA®, a student movement active on campus at hundreds of universities, colleges and schools of nursing in the United States of America, and a member movement of the International Fellowship of Evangelical Students. For information about local and regional activities, write Public Relations Dept., InterVarsity Christian Fellowship/USA, 6400 Schroeder Rd., P.O. Box 7895, Madison, WI 53707-7895.

Cover illustration: Hero of Faith, Florence Nightingale. World Christian Fellowship stained glass window in The Upper Room Chapel, Nashville, Tennessee. Used by permission of The Upper Room Chapel.

ISBN 0-8308-1598-8

Printed in the United States of America ♾

Library of Congress Cataloging-in-Publication Data has been requested.

Shelly, Judith Allen.
Called to care: a Christian theology of nursing/Judith Allen Shelly & Arlene B. Miller.
p. cm.
Includes bibliographical references and indexes.
ISBN 0-8308-1598-8 (pbk.: alk. paper)
1. Nursing—Religious aspects—Christianity. 2. Nursing—Philosophy. 3. Christian life. I. Miller, Arlene B., 1935- .
II. Title.
RT85.2.S538 1999
610.73'01—dc21

99-10868
CIP

24 23 22 21 19 18 17 16 15 14 13 12 11 10 9 8 7 6 5
17 16 15 14 13 12 11 10 09 08 07 06 05 04 03

Preface

This book began as a conversation. It was the summer of 1984 at the Nurses Christian Fellowship conference in Burton, Ohio. Although we (Arlene and Judy) had heard about one another for several years, this was the first time we had actually met. We began to talk about our hopes and dreams for nursing—and our concerns. We concluded the conversation by agreeing that, if trends continued as they were, nursing as we knew it would cease to exist in ten years. Then we prayed for the profession we both loved.

We sensed a deep kindred spirit. Most of the concerns we shared had been quickly dismissed by colleagues when we expressed them in other settings. What a relief to find another person who shared the vision! The conversation grew into a friendship, and we kept talking. We observed and discussed nursing trends. We watched paradigms shift—both economic and philosophical. We studied changing values in nursing. To a great extent, nursing as we knew it *did* cease to exist. In 1993 we coauthored *Values in Conflict: Christian Nursing in a Changing Profession;* but even before that manuscript was off the press, we sensed that it was only the beginning. We immediately began thinking about another book on the theological foundations of nursing.

We believe that nurses cannot separate our professional roles from our profession of faith—regardless of what our culture tells us about keeping religion private. Furthermore, we are convinced that Christian faith is the very heart of nursing theory and practice. This book is addressed primarily to nurses who call themselves Christians and are trying to think through the implications of that commitment in their professional lives. We hope that others will also find it helpful.

The book is organized around the nursing metaparadigm. We begin with a brief overview in chapters 1—3, then carefully examine and expand each concept in the metaparadigm—the person (chaps. 4—6), the environment (chaps. 7—9), health (chaps. 10—12) and nursing practice (chaps. 13—15)—identifying the implications of the biblical worldview as it relates to each area. We will also continually revisit the effects of modernism and postmodernism as they impinge on each concept. Since their influence is complex and pervasive, it may seem as if we are beating the same drum over and over. Our intent, however, is to demonstrate the subtle ways in which our Christian worldview can shift to other paradigms as we move from one concept to another.

Over the years, others have joined the conversation. Sharon Fish, Jim Sire, Phyllis Karns and Verna Carson helped us think about and refine the concepts discussed in this book. We have presented the basic content of the book in Christian and secular professional conferences in the United States, Hong Kong, Taiwan, Korea and the Netherlands—and heard lively responses. We particularly appreciate our friends in Korea who helped us better understand *ki* energy: Susie Kim, Chung Nam Kim, Lee Won Hee and Carol Findlay. Arlene has taught the material to baccalaureate nursing students, refining it each year. Judy has taught it in a graduate course and written about it in *Journal of Christian Nursing* editorials and other professional-journal articles. Each time, the material took clearer shape. In the process of writing the book, we both completed doctorates, and we are deeply grateful to our professors—including those who disagreed with and challenged us.

Mary Thompson, national director of Nurses Christian Fellowship, and Sandra Jamison, Chair of the Nursing Department at Messiah College—our bosses—demonstrated utmost patience with us as the project dragged on to four years. They guarded our time and facilitated our work in every way possible. Sandy also served as a dissertation committee member for Judy.

Arlene received two faculty grants from Messiah College. Judy received funding from the Huston Foundation, Tenth Presbyterian Church, Narberth Presbyterian Church and many faithful individuals. To each we are deeply grateful.

We are also thankful for our friends and family who encouraged, supported and put up with us in this long, often tedious process. Many of them could not understand what we were talking about, but they sensed it was important, so they prayed for us and loved us anyhow. Special thanks go to Judy's husband, Jim, and children, Janell and Jon. And last, but not least, we want to thank Janice Bridgman, who dropped in from New Zealand to pull weeds, paint woodwork and hang wallpaper so we could finish the task.

Part One

Introduction

1

Caring & the Christian Story

CHRISTINE, AN EMERGENCY-DEPARTMENT STAFF NURSE IN AN inner-city hospital, saw two little boys running out of the men's room shouting, "Someone's lying on the floor in there!" Rushing in to investigate, she found a leather-coated man of about thirty lying face down on the floor, cyanotic. She felt a pulse—but no breath. Christine knew he was most likely an overdosed intravenous drug user and HIV-positive, but when help seemed long in coming, she began mouth-to-mouth resuscitation in spite of her fears. Afterward her colleagues said she had been irresponsible. But all Christine could think about was, *If Jesus lived today, would he sit among the HIV-positive and love them?*[1]

Rosene, a nurse in an extended-care facility, felt repulsed at first by the "concentrated assemblage of helpless humanity" that surrounded her. But then she prayerfully determined that she would get to know her patients and see in each one the image of God. She gradually began to enjoy the people in her care.[2]

Marsha, caring for an obscenity-shouting, combative drug abuser, looked into his eyes and saw a person whom God loved.[3]

Mother Teresa saw Jesus in the sick and dying of Calcutta and took them in to comfort and care for them.

Joy, an American nurse living in Turkey, saw starving babies in an orphanage and organized an ongoing project to provide them with nourishing formula.[4]

What common thread weaves throughout these stories? Each of the nurses responded to her patients from a theological commitment. They saw those in their care as valuable human beings who reflected the image of God. They saw hope in the midst of hopeless situations. They viewed health as a holistic concept that radiates from a vital relationship with God and includes physical integrity, emotional stability and participation in the life of the community. They were motivated by the desire to share the love of God, which they had personally experienced, and they saw nursing as compassionate service to God and their neighbors.

How does what we believe affect the health care we provide? Is there a relationship between the way a society understands the nature of God and the type of health care that develops in that society? We will argue that there is a direct relationship and that if the faith perspective changes, health care practices will change. In fact, we are living in the midst of such changes in North America right now.

Nursing developed out of a Christian worldview. It is important to see that *the changes we are experiencing stem from a growing paradigm shift in our culture.* To fully appreciate this shift, we must first look at who we are and how nursing developed in the first place.

How Did We Get Here?

Optimism ran high in mid-nineteenth-century England. With the rise of empiricism, in which all knowledge is derived from experience, science blossomed and gave rise to high hopes for conquering drudgery and disease. Florence Nightingale went to the Crimea, and by applying good principles of sanitation she made a major difference in the death rate of British soldiers (from 42 percent to 2 percent). But the spectacular success of science and high hopes of the philosophers had an unsettling effect on the common people—and that troubled Nightingale.

She wrote to her friend John Stuart Mill, "Many years ago, I had a large and very curious acquaintance among the artisans of the North of England and of London. I learned that they were without any religion whatever—though diligently seeking after one, principally in Comte and his school. Any return to what is called Christianity appeared impossible."[5] The people were turning to empiricism and becoming atheists.

At the same time, corruption and controversy filled the Church of England. While the church could be rigid in its outward requirements, it tended to be elitist and hypocritical in practice. In the light of the positivism of science and philosophy and the negativism of the church, many of the common people became disillusioned and simply dropped out.

Florence Nightingale seemed most concerned about the ethical implications of religious belief. In her book *Suggestions for Thought* she attempted to develop an alternative concept of God that would appeal to the disenchanted "artisans" (merchants and craftsmen) so they would have a basis for morality. Her theology was far from orthodox—she dismissed the incarnation, the Trinity and the atonement as "abortions of a comprehension of God's plan."[6] However, she considered herself a Christian and her work a "call from God."[7]

The Enlightenment brought major changes in science beginning with René Descartes (1596-1650) and his elevation of human reason. The move toward modern science began with British physicist Isaac Newton's *Mathematical Principles of Natural Philosophy* (1687), in which he postulated that mathematical physics could explain the whole of the physical universe (the "mechanical world"). John Locke (1632-1704) and George Berkeley (1685-1753) continued this move to empiricism, retaining a somewhat Christian flavor that resulted in theological deism.

The twentieth century brought another set of philosophical and theological problems into the picture. New philosophers built on the foundations laid by empiricism, then began tearing them down. The results were nihilism, existentialism and eventually postmodernism. This philosophical ferment laid the foundation for the tension we face in nursing today.

Do the philosophical and theological underpinnings of nursing really matter? Absolutely! For just as Florence Nightingale observed that the common people in her day were becoming atheists and thereby losing their basis for ethical behavior, people today are affected by the philosophies of our time. Optimism and progress do not seem to work. But at the same time, we have grown comfortable with the benefits of technology. The desperate scramblings of twentieth-century theologians to communicate the gospel to a modern generation led to liberalism and disillusionment. The monism of Eastern spirituality grows increasingly attractive to a discouraged and alienated age. The spirit of service and compassion that once motivated nurses has evolved into a professionalism that demands power, status and appropriate compensation. We see the effects in a health care system controlled by the bottom line and a desperate grasping for alternative approaches to healing.

The Enlightenment deluded us into thinking that what we believe does not affect what we do—that we can keep our faith and our nursing work in separate boxes. Postmodernism restores the integration, but it insists that while my truth is important to me, I cannot impose it on you. Both assume that we can function in the public square without a moral basis for our community life. While the general public may not be confronted with the reality of this notion on a regular basis, in nursing we cannot escape it. We see the problem with separating faith and ethics every time we deal with crucial human situations—not only the big problems of abortion and euthanasia but even the daily matters of providing responsible nursing care.

What Is Nursing?

In recent history nursing has been closely associated with medicine and often confused with the medical profession; however, nursing and medicine are two distinct professions with very different histories. Western medicine developed out of a Greek, and later Cartesian, body-mind dualism that viewed the body as object.[8] The role of the nurse, however, grew out of a Christian understanding of the human person as created in the image of God and viewed the body as a living unity and the "temple of the Holy Spirit" (1 Cor 3:16).

Medicine has traditionally focused on the scientific dimension of the human body, relegating the spiritual and psychosocial dimensions to religion and psychology. The uniqueness of nursing is its emphasis on caring for the whole person as embodied. It is defined as both an art and a science. Anne

Bishop and Jack Scudder insist that nursing is neither an art nor a science but a *practice* that draws on both the arts and sciences.[9] Nursing, even in our most scientifically oriented periods, has always been concerned with the whole person. Nurse theorist Patricia Benner asserts,

> Nurses deal with not only normality and pathophysiology but also with the lived social and skilled body in promoting health, growth, and development and in caring for the sick and dying.[10]

In other words, nurses work from an understanding of the self as embodied and are concerned with how we relate to one another and function in the world through our bodies.

The classic definition of nursing, developed by theorist Virginia Henderson and adopted by the International Council of Nurses, states:

> The unique function of the nurse is to assist the individual, sick or well, in the performance of those activities contributing to health or its recovery (or to peaceful death) that he would perform unaided if he had the necessary strength, will or knowledge. And to do this in such a way as to help him gain independence as rapidly as possible.[11]

Henderson further elaborates by listing fourteen activities that a nurse assists patients to perform.[12] Eight of these activities pertain directly to bodily functions. The remaining six relate to safety and finding meaning and purpose in life—enabling the embodied person to function in relation to other people and the environment in a healthy way.

More recent definitions, while not completely denying the need for physical care, reflect a growing paradigm shift by focusing more on the psychosocial aspects of care and less on the physical. For example, Martha Rogers states, "Professional practice in nursing seeks to promote symphonic interaction between man and environment, to strengthen the coherence and integrity of the human field and to direct and redirect patterning of the human and environmental fields for the realization of maximum health potential."[13]

Jean Watson asserts, "At its most basic level nursing is a human, caring, relational profession. . . . Caring in nursing is a 'human mode of being'; caring is a basic way of 'being-in-the-world' and creates both self and world."[14]

Rosemarie Rizzo Parse further expands this approach to nursing: "The nurse centers with the universe, prepares, and approaches the other, attending intensely to the meaning of the moment being lived by the person or family."[15]

With the present tumultuous change in the health care system, nursing struggles to redefine itself. While theorists move toward the psychosocial and ethereal, practitioners are positioning themselves for professional survival. Both teeter on a precipice, in peril of losing the true essence of nursing entirely. The former are looking more like shamans and the latter like physician-technicians. Neither embraces the full concept of *nurse* that grew out of the Christian gospel.

We will define Christian nursing as *a ministry of compassionate care for the whole person, in response to God's grace toward a sinful world, which aims to foster optimum health* (shalom) *and bring comfort in suffering and death for anyone in need.*

A Brief History of Nursing

Although some forms of health care were provided in ancient cultures,[16] nurse historian Patricia Donahue states, "The history of nursing first becomes continuous with the beginning of Christianity."[17] Nurse historians Dolan, Fitzpatrick and Herrmann state,

> The teachings and example of Jesus Christ had a profound influence on the emergence of gifted nurse leadership as well as on the expansion of the role of nurses. Christ stressed the need to love God and one's neighbor. The first organized group of nurses was established as a direct response to His example and challenge.[18]

The impetus for this movement came when the first-century Christians began to teach that all believers were ministers who were to care for the poor, the sick and the disenfranchised (Mt 25:31-46; Heb 13:1-3; Jas 1:27; 1 Pet 2:9). As the churches grew, they appointed deacons to care for the needy within the church.[19] Eventually, more men and women were added to the roll of deacons, and their designated responsibilities grew to include caring for the sick.[20] Phoebe, the deacon mentioned in Romans 16:1-2, is often considered the first visiting nurse.[21]

By the third century, organized groups of deaconesses were caring for the sick, insane and lepers in the community.[22] In the fourth century the church began establishing hospitals. Most of these hospitals did not have a physician; they were staffed by nurses. There were several periods when the early church did not condone the practice of medicine, which they viewed as a pagan art.[23] Nurse historians Lavinia Dock and Isabel Stewart state,

> The age-old custom of hospitality ... was practiced with religious fervor by the early Christians. . . . Their houses were opened wide to every afflicted applicant and, not satisfied with receiving needy ones, the deacons, men and women alike, went out to search and bring them in.[24]

Nursing in the Middle Ages centered in monasteries. Women who wanted to serve God and care for the sick joined together in monastic orders. In the late Middle Ages, the Knights Hospitallers of St. John, a military nursing order, built a hospital in Jerusalem, as well as others along the route of the Crusades. While the original intent was to care for pilgrims to Jerusalem, they also cared for Muslims, Jews and Christian crusaders.[25]

The Renaissance through the eighteenth century brought a dark period in the history of nursing. As Catholic religious orders were disbanded or suppressed in Protestant countries, hospitals deteriorated. Nursing ceased to be a public role; it moved out of the church and into the home. However, some religious orders in southern Europe continued providing nursing care, including those established by St. Francis de Sales (1567-1662) and St. Vincent de Paul (1576-1669).[26] However, care deteriorated even among the religious orders as nuns were not allowed to touch any part of the human body except the head and extremities and were often forced to work twenty-four-hour days.[27]

By the nineteenth century, except for a few nursing orders of nuns, nursing was disorganized and corrupt. Dolan et al. describe hospitals in Philadelphia in 1884:

> Hospital patients were penniless folk, usually homeless and friendless. In most of the city hospitals the nursing was done by inmates usually

over 50 years old, many being 70 or 80. . . . There was practically no night nursing, except for the "night watchers" provided for women in childbirth and the dying.[28]

Charles Dickens portrayed nineteenth-century nursing in the character of Sairey Gamp in his novel *Martin Chuzzlewit*.[29] A self-seeking alcoholic, Gamp has become the symbol of nursing at its worst. Dickens focused public attention on the nursing care being provided by alcoholics, prostitutes and women who were uncaring and immoral.

Reform again came through the work of the Christian church. Elizabeth Seton established the Widow's Society in New York to care for poor women in their homes—to nurse and comfort them. She later joined the Catholic church and eventually established the Sisters of Charity at Emmitsburg, Maryland. Mother Mary Catherine McAuley founded the Sisters of Mercy, who ministered to the poor and sick in Dublin, Ireland, and eventually spread to other countries, including the United States. Elizabeth Fry, an American Quaker in London, began a campaign of prison reform that eventually developed into the Society of Protestant Sisters of Charity, whose primary objective was to supply nurses for the sick of all classes in their homes.[30]

Fry had a strong influence on a German Lutheran pastor, Theodor Fliedner, and his wife, Frederika. Seeing the pressing needs of the poor and the sick in their community, the Fliedners decided that the church must care for these people. They turned a little garden house into a home for outcast girls and eventually organized a community of deaconesses to visit and nurse the sick in their homes. That experiment quickly grew into the Kaiserswerth Institute for the Training of Deaconesses, with a huge complex of buildings, including a hospital, and educational programs for nurses and teachers.[31]

About the same time, a young woman in England, Florence Nightingale, felt God calling her to future service. She responded to that call by becoming a nurse, studying first at the Kaiserswerth Institute, then at Catholic hospitals in Paris. Nightingale went on to single-handedly reform nursing, bringing it back to its Christian roots and setting high educational and practice standards.[32] However, her theological influence also set the stage for an ongoing struggle between those of her followers who wanted to be viewed as "professional" and those who understood nursing as a calling from God—a conflict Nightingale herself did not envision.

About this same period, churches in Europe and the United States began establishing hospitals with schools of nursing. William Passavant, a Lutheran pastor and pioneer in hospital development, visited Kaiserswerth and brought deaconesses to Pittsburgh, Pennsylvania, to staff his first hospital.

The growing division between "professional nurses" and deaconesses was already evident at this time. Passavant described the tension between Christian service and professionalism in an address given in 1899:

> The deaconess has a Biblical office, the nurse a worldly vocation. The one serves through love; the other for her support. In the one case we have an exercise of charity as wide in extent as the sufferings and misery of mankind; in the other, a usefulness circumscribed by the narrow circle of obedient help given to the physicians and surgeons. Above all, the deaconess cares for the body in order to reach the soul. She works for eternity. The trained nurse, like the man whose vocation brings him to the sick-bed, is, as a rule, quite content to pass by unnoticed the possibilities of an eternal future in the demands of the present welfare of the patient.[33]

Influential nursing leaders at the turn of the century railed against the idea of nursing as a religious calling for several reasons.[34] British empiricism left many thinking people of the time disillusioned with the church and placing their hopes in science. Also, most nurses in the religious orders and deaconess communities worked under oppressive conditions, resulting in chronic fatigue and a high mortality rate among nurses.[35]

At the same time, the American social context included a strong sense of progress and an assumption that freedom and democracy would eventually create a pure, rational society. But rapid industrialization had left society with a loss of community and large populations of disenfranchised poor. Upper-middle-class women, as keepers of the culture's mores and unable to hold paying jobs, became social reformers. Out of these developments public health nursing arose. Nurse historian Diane Hamilton comments about these nurse reformers ("inventors"):

> Thus, both nursing and religion, if pursued compassionately, healed wounded minds, bodies, and spirits. Although the nurse inventors intended an unyielding boundary between religion and nursing, the kindred missions of religion and nursing rendered the boundary translucent. They envisioned that secular nursing would emulate the values of the religious sisters without accepting their rules, regulations, and cloistered life. Compassion, once associated with God's authority, would, according to the nurse inventors, be replaced with compassion based on commitment to the authority of humanity and its social progress.[36]

Other nursing leaders during the same period insisted that the intimacy inherent in nursing practice required religious goodness, credulity, discipline and obedience. Charlotte Aikens, in a 1924 nursing ethics text, acknowledged "religion" (defined as "the relation which an individual fixes between his soul and his God") as the basis for nursing ethics.[37] Rebecca McNeill wrote in the *American Journal of Nursing* in 1910 that the "ideal nurse" must be a Christian.[38]

Adding to the tension between the secular and religious influences in nursing was the common practice of deaconess hospitals' establishing schools of nursing based on the Nightingale system, so that, until the establishment of baccalaureate nursing programs, the two philosophies—service and professionalism—developed side by side. As a baccalaureate nursing student in the early sixties, I (Judy) felt caught in the middle of this tension. When I wrote a class paper for a course in nursing leadership, I chose to defend the idea of *service*. In the process, I raised the ire of my instructor.

While professional nursing grew in Western countries, the evangelical missionary movement also began. Early missionaries went to Asia and Africa, communicating the gospel primarily through education and health care. Florence Nightingale also sent out "missioners" to all English-speaking countries.[39] Although they determined to be secular, most drew their motivation from Christian faith and often worked through religious orders or mission hospitals. As missionary activity spread around the world, nursing worldwide could trace its roots to Florence Nightingale and a Christian worldview.

Nursing Today

With the current rise of alternative spiritualities among nursing leaders, revisionist approaches to nursing history have attempted to bypass the Christian roots of nursing. More recent nursing histories look instead to animistic "medicine men and women" and shamans, Greek and Roman goddesses, Egyptian priestesses, Ayuvedic medicine, and healing traditions based on *chi* energy.[40]

The practical result of these approaches seems to be a move away from the physical care of the body.[41] Increasingly, nursing as practiced by advocates of alternative healing occurs more in the mind and less with hands-on physical care. While "caring" is taught, it is more of a detached presence than a doing of those things that communicate compassion.[42]

At the same time nursing is facing a major restructuring and redefinition based on bottom-line economics. American Nurses Association research has indicated that the reduction of registered nurses in hospitals is causing unsafe conditions for some patients. The most frequently reported explanations for the nurse cutbacks were economic reasons.[43]

Not only does the health care industry want to streamline the work force to save money, but some nurses themselves seem to be more motivated by economic considerations. Nurse educator Susan Stocker writes:

> I'm seeing an increasing number of students who are not entering nursing for the same reasons you and I did. They don't have a caring attitude. They have a goal and that goal is to get a job that pays a decent wage. The end. What impact will that have on the professional organization and the profession?[44]

Why are we in nursing? Is it only to earn a decent wage? Are we hoping to gain power and prestige or academic status? While nurses have traditionally entered nursing to serve God and care for the sick, those motivations seem to be rapidly changing. Too many nurses start lining up at the time clock to punch out while patient call lights flash. Others retreat to academia to avoid the unpleasant tasks of staff nursing.

Tanya, a senior in a nursing program where students were allowed to choose their clinical areas, smugly related that she had managed to arrange all of her clinical experience in psychiatric settings. She had never done any physical care. When asked how she hoped to function as a graduate nurse, she adamantly stated, "I didn't go into nursing to carry bedpans."

Jesus Christ has called us to a different vision for nursing. He touched lepers (Lk 5). He applied mud compresses (Jn 9:6). He washed feet (Jn 13). Jesus clearly proclaimed, "Whoever wishes to become great among you must be your servant, and whoever wishes to be first among you must be slave of all. For the Son of Man came not to be served but to serve, and to give his life a ransom for many" (Mk 10:43-45).

As Jesus began his ministry he proclaimed:

> The Spirit of the Lord is upon me,
>   because he has anointed me
>   to bring good news to the poor.
> He has sent me to proclaim release to the
>   captives
>   and recovery of sight to the blind,
>   to let the oppressed go free,
>   to proclaim the year of the Lord's favor.
>   (Lk 4:18-19)

Throughout the Gospels, physical healing was intimately linked with the proclamation of the gospel. Jesus sent his followers out with instructions to heal the sick and to tell them, "The kingdom of God has come near to you" (Lk 10:9). He underlined our responsibility to provide physical care by explaining in Matthew 25:

> I was hungry and you gave me food, I was thirsty and you gave me something to drink, I was a stranger and you welcomed me, I was naked and you gave me clothing, I was sick and you took care of me.

. . . Truly I tell you, just as you did it to one of the least of these who are members of my family, you did it to me.

However, he did not stop there. Throughout the Gospels we see how the ultimate purpose for physical healing was to restore people to a vital relationship with God and the community.

If that is the case, nursing cannot work toward the goal of health without including the clear proclamation of the gospel, as well as providing physical care with a servant attitude. Nursing as a vocation, or *calling*, from God, must return to its roots in the church and Christian faith in order to work toward the goal of true health. Furthermore, if we hope to maintain a strong Christian worldview in nursing, our faith must be nurtured in a Christian community and informed by a clear theology. True nursing cannot be divorced from the Christian story.

2

Revolution in the Nursing Paradigm

SONJA FACED A DILEMMA. WORKING ON A LARGE AIDS UNIT over several years, she grew to care deeply for the men and women who were frequently readmitted as a result of their immunosuppression. She grieved when they died, and she recommitted herself to making the lives of other patients as comfortable as possible during their last days. Her sense of being called by the Lord gave her strength for what was often exhausting work.

Increasingly, however, Sonja began to think that the option of physician-assisted suicide made sense for her patients. Many on her unit were seeking the help of organizations encouraging "the right to die" as a way of ending their prolonged suffering. Some of her colleagues argued that helping these patients end their lives was an act of compassion. Sonja felt confused. She knew that she could not deliberately end the life of anyone in her care. Yet watching her patients suffer moved her to consider helping them contact someone for information about suicide as an option. Although this alternative violated all that she had learned in nursing school about care for the dying, recent articles in nursing journals argued for the right of patients to control their own deaths, dying when they chose to do so.

Maria faced another dilemma when she returned to school for a master's degree and took a required course in nursing theory. Like many of her fellow classmates in undergraduate school, she had viewed nursing theory as one of the subjects to be endured on the way to "real nursing." Now, however, she was trying to see some practical implications in it.

The changes in how nurses thought about nursing over the years intrigued her. Florence Nightingale focused on natural laws and the environment; then Virginia Henderson saw nurses acting as substitutes to meet patients' needs when they could not do it themselves. Martha Rogers began to view patients as energy fields within larger energy fields. Because Maria was a deeply committed Christian, she wondered about the connection between the theories she was studying and her faith.

One professor suggested that she read the creation story in Genesis, substituting the word "energy" for "God." Upon trying it she realized that it undermined her understanding of the Christian God, who reveals himself as personal and loving. Over and over throughout the Scriptures God speaks of wanting to dwell with his people, of wanting to be their God and to have them belong to him. This was the language of love and commitment. Energy, the language of physics, was so impersonal.

Karen, a junior nursing student at a large university, faced another dilemma. One of her favorite instructors was teaching a popular elective course in alternative healing, so Karen enthusiastically signed up for it. She hoped to learn new ways to comfort patients. As the weeks went by, however, she began to feel uncomfortable with what she was learning. For example, the professor told the class that she considered herself a witch and that some of the healing methods she taught were "white witchcraft." She encouraged students to chant formulas and burn candles as part of the healing process. She also taught that the Christian church had persecuted witches in order to retain its power over women. During a field trip to a center for therapeutic touch, the instructor encouraged students to take off their clothes as a way to break down barriers between themselves. Karen struggled with knowing what to do. What was happening?[1]

Sonja, Maria and Karen are not alone in their bewilderment. Nursing—reflecting changes in the larger Western culture—is undergoing major shifts in its thinking and practice. The foundations of nursing itself are being questioned. What is nursing about? What should be the goals of nursing?

What is science in nursing? How can these questions be answered?

The Beginnings of Nursing Theory

Until nursing education moved from hospital-based apprentice programs to the academic setting, there was little formal analysis of such matters. Nightingale's concern for a well-ordered environment was taken for granted, and much of nursing focused around keeping things clean. During the early 1900s, hospitals were staffed by nursing students who worked long hours and studied when they could. After graduation nurses went into either private-duty or public health nursing. Most women in nursing were motivated by Christian values of compassion and service. Nurses saw themselves, for the most part, as assistants to physicians. There was little time or inclination to develop concepts and philosophies of nursing.

As nursing education moved into academia, the need developed to establish a body of knowledge unique to nursing. Because nursing entered the academy through science departments, such knowledge was to be based on research. Scientific research required theories. Serious efforts in theory development began in the 1950s and proliferated in the 1960s and 1970s. Virginia Henderson articulated her famous definition of nursing in 1961 in a pamphlet published by the International Council of Nurses.[2]

Because nursing entered the university through the door of natural science, nursing theories took on characteristics of naturalism. They were couched in cause-and-effect language, often with elaborate diagrams showing complex relationships between concepts. Many theorists of this era were psychiatric nurses, so their theories focused on the nurse-patient relationship.[3] Even these were framed in naturalistic language of analysis and cause and effect, although in a more personal tone.

Early nursing theories reflect the positivistic philosophy of science prevalent in the university.[4] According to positivism, it is possible to gain true knowledge of reality (what actually exists) through the processes of theory development and testing. The scientific community accepts theories insofar as they seem to correspond with reality. Nurses hoped that through this process of theory testing and refinement they would progressively build the body of knowledge needed for both patient care and credibility in academia.

Early in this era (1952), the journal *Nursing Research* began to disseminate the findings of researchers. Great optimism among nurses in academia characterized this period.

Meanwhile nurses practicing at the bedside felt little actual impact from either nursing theories or nursing research. They did, however, experience the impact of new medical technology in the development of critical care units, advances in surgery and new approaches to emergency treatment. But these practicing nurses always knew that there was more to nursing than technology. They were often in awe of the inner strength of their patients as they struggled with overwhelming illnesses, sometimes recovering, sometimes dying. Nurses understood the power of their relationships with patients to encourage and give hope.

Then in 1962 Thomas Kuhn published *The Structure of Scientific Revolutions,* in which he challenged the prevailing assumption that science was value-free. Kuhn is often misread as implying that reality exists only in human perception. What he does say is that while our perception and values shape our understanding of reality, eventually "reality fights back," telling us that our theories are incorrect. In other words the facts no longer fit the theory.[5] A new paradigm, or way of interpreting experience, is sought. He denies, however, that progress in science means drawing us closer to "some goal set by nature in advance."[6]

Since Kuhn published his book, nurse thinkers, along with many in the social and natural sciences, have wrestled with questions about the nature of science itself. Nursing theory textbooks now include chapters on the philosophy of science,[7] asking questions such as *What is truth? What is theory?* They are also asking even more basic questions such as *Does reality exist beyond our perceptions, and, if it does, can we know anything at all about it? What is the scientific method?* The debate rages in every field of study. Nurses have an advantage that many others are not given—the patients we face every time we work. If the facts do not fit our theories, we get rapid feedback.

However, the other side of Kuhn's argument is that changing our thinking does not come to us easily, either as individuals or as a community of thinkers and practitioners. He likens such changes to a conversion, something that one *experiences*. They are not brought about by logical argument. The old ways of interpreting our experiences with patients continue to guide us until we suddenly see the facts in a new way.

Conversion to a New Paradigm

Nursing is currently undergoing such a conversion experience. For many years nurses have known intuitively that there was more about ourselves and our patients than could be explained within naturalistic scientific theories.[8] Every day we experience life, death, tragedy, birth and suffering. How often patients press us with questions. "Why did my baby die?" "How can I live with a body that can't move or feel?" How often have we stood dumb before these cries? Our theories were impotent to help us. The naturalistic scientific theories told us about physiology and pathology. The psychosocial nursing theories told us to listen, to feel with, to support and encourage our patients. But we found ourselves powerless in the end. Many of us turned to our faith to help us, and for most nurses that was Christian faith.

Then in 1970 Martha Rogers published her little text *An Introduction to the Theoretical Basis of Nursing*.[9] Because her work was so radically different, many dismissed both the book and Rogers herself. Few understood what she was saying, and even fewer grasped the significance of what she was doing for nursing.[10] What she did was open possibilities for new ways of thinking about nursing. Rogers continued using the impersonal language of physics—energy, field theory, simultaneity—to describe the intangible in nursing, but she loaded these words with new meaning. Other nursing theorists who followed began to explore new approaches to nursing theory and science, such as phenomenology and existentialism, and to use the language of *spirit, consciousness* and *goddess*.[11]

In the 1994 edition of her textbook on nursing theory, Barbara Stevens Barnum notes the polarity between the older and the newer nursing theories. The older nursing process theories are associated with taxonomies and quantitative measures, whereas the new holistic theories use more qualitative measures and softer phenomena.[12]

Both nursing education and practice are feeling the impact of the shift from the old to the new approaches. This shift—or revolution, according to

Kuhn—is what Sonja, Maria and Karen, who were introduced at the beginning of this chapter, are experiencing. The shift affects not merely our thinking about nursing but also our nursing interventions and the way we make ethical decisions.

The polarity Barnum notes is particularly wide when it comes to how we develop nursing knowledge. Two opposing and irreconcilable ontologies (views of reality) underlie the old and the new paradigms: realism and conceptualism.[13] Barnum writes:

> In realism, one believes that the world exists "out there," independent of the knower. Research and theory seek to discover and explain the nature of that external reality. . . . In conceptualism, reality does not exist independent of the knower. Invention, rather than discovery, is the dominant mode of knowing reality. The two concepts are the extreme poles, with all sorts of variations on the continuum that spans them.[14]

Barnum, like many other nurse thinkers, advocates a live-and-let-live approach between these two paradigms in nursing, arguing that both have something to contribute. If Kuhn is correct in his analysis, however, conversation between those using different paradigms is not possible. The struggle between them will continue until the new paradigm succeeds the old.[15]

Some nurse thinkers debate the question at the level of philosophy and science.[16] Margretta Styles sees the need for nursing to be guided by a unity of science based on philosophy, to clarify "what we *should* be and to include in professionalization such themes as commitment, personal motivation, and self-actualization as well as scientific discovery."[17]

While we agree that naturalistic theories alone are much too narrow for nursing, we also think that there are serious problems with many of the newer approaches. We agree with Styles that the issue is much more fundamental. It lies with our ultimate view of life, the philosophy of nursing. We appreciate the new openness to spirituality—but we believe that there is a far deeper concern than merely adding religion and spirituality, as if they were the missing parts that will slack the hunger for meaning not addressed in naturalistic theories. What is happening in nursing (and in our larger culture) is a major shift from one worldview to another. The new theories in nursing reflect this shift. It is at the worldview level that we must begin.

Beginning with Worldviews

Until recently the term *worldview* was part of the technical language of philosophers and anthropologists. Philosophers refer to worldview when they mean the basic assumptions that underlie a system of thought. Anthropologists use the term in a broader way to identify not only the wellsprings of our thinking but our way of life as well. "It shapes and integrates our various fields of knowledge from theology, anthropology, and missions to physics and the culinary arts. Worldview governs everyday behavior"[18] (Mt 6:8; 7:11; Lk 12:32). "Worldviews are the most fundamental and encompassing views of reality shared by a people in a culture. A worldview incorporates assumptions about the nature of things—about the 'givens' of reality"[19] (Heb 4:15). "They are made up of the categories, values, and assumptions we use to examine our world."[20] Worldviews provide the cultural lenses that shape how we see the world, and they give meaning to life, both personally and for humanity as a whole.

Because a worldview is so overarching, it can integrate many theories from different aspects of life and help us see how they may complement each other. But when theories reflect very different worldviews, they will conflict with one another. Ultimately, differing worldviews cannot be reconciled; either one or the other gives us a truer picture of reality.

The Modern Western Worldview

Scholars trace some themes of the worldview governing modern Western culture back to the Indo-European culture of the third millennium B.C. According to anthropologist Paul Hiebert, this worldview in its various forms undergirded the religions of Babylon, Sumer, Canaan, Greece, India and Germany, among others.

In this worldview good and evil are two independent entities locked in eternal conflict. In this battle, the ultimate good is order and freedom, and to achieve this one side or the other must gain control. The ultimate evil is chaos and enslavement. Given this dualism, all reality is divided into two camps and the line between them is sharp. We see this in our American tendency to categorize in opposites: good-bad, big-small, sweet-sour, success-failure, and truth-falsehood.[21]

Dualism[22] in modern thinking was reinforced by the introduction of Greek thinking into Western culture during the Renaissance when the writings of Plato and Aristotle were once again being read. Medieval Christianity, strongly influenced by Greek thinking, drew a sharp line between spirit and matter. Theologians saw matter and the world as inherently evil, spirit and heaven as good. They drew a sharp distinction between the natural and the supernatural. Their focus was the supernatural realm of God, Satan, angels, demons, heaven, hell, sin, salvation and miracles.

During the Renaissance, thinkers turned to the natural world of humans, animals, plants and matter. They began to see the world as autonomous, operating according to natural laws. Their hope was that the newly developing science would enable them to understand these laws and use them to solve practical human problems.[23] While early scientists saw the world as an orderly creation dependent on God for its existence, increasingly people thought of God as distant. Humans were responsible to solve their own problems. This view eventually led to the modern secularism that effectively eliminates God from public life.

Placing human beings and human concerns above God and what he wants for us is the result of this secularism. During the Renaissance, Machiavelli called on people to forget about salvation and focus on enjoying life here and now on the earth. Personal happiness, comfort and property became the central goals of Western culture, and science was seen as the means to achieve them.[24] However, being at the top of the universe is a lonely position, and eventually many modern people wondered what life is all about. Hiebert points out that when science was applied to human beings it reduced them, made them less than human.

[People were seen as] animals ruled by needs and irrational drives (Freudian psychology), as stimulus-response machines (behavioral psychology), or as robots programmed by their societies and cultures (sociology and anthropology). God was gone, but so was the human soul. There was no real meaning in human life.[25]

While the modern worldview retains these dualistic themes inherited from the ancient Indo-Europeans and Greeks, it has also been influenced by Hebrew and Christian thinking. The Bible has given the Western world its strong emphasis on the value of the individual person who is not to be lost within the group. The biblical teaching that life has its source in God and that humans are created with the capacity to relate to God in a personal way has supported our respect for each person. The creation story undergirds our belief that creation is orderly and that the "laws" of nature can be discerned by science. Westerners get the idea of history as going somewhere to a climax, rather than in endless natural cycles, from the biblical story of God acting in history and finally bringing it to a conclusion. Biblical values of love and justice have shaped Western ethics.

Today many are dismissing the modern worldview as having been tried and found wanting, seeing it as causing alienation from the world of the spirit. Some see Christianity as part of the problem, because it has become so intertwined with the modern worldview. Nevertheless, its themes are still powerful in our culture even though they are reinterpreted on a secular basis. Both Christianity and Indo-European and Greek dualism have under-girded the rise of modern science and the concept of progress associated with it.

The Postmodern Worldview

Many writers are arguing that we now live in a postmodern world.[26] Despite the powerful benefits of science, there is increasing recognition that science cannot give meaning to life. Many scientists are themselves rejecting the dualism that divorces spiritual from material realities and separates values from scientific objectivity. Social scientists and health care professionals are calling for a more holistic view that brings humans into harmony with their environment. Others, rejecting hierarchy and competition, are calling for more inclusive global cooperation.

The newer theorists of nursing reflect this postmodern worldview: Patricia Benner, Joyce Fitzpatrick, Margaret Newman, Rosemarie Rizzo Parse, Martha E. Rogers and Jean Watson. Each of these thinkers is quite different in her approach, but each is calling for something beyond the mechanistic, natural-science approach to nursing. A new nursing paradigm is needed.

Many of the New Paradigm theories are based on an assumption that the world is made up of an impersonal energy that can be manipulated and controlled.[27] These theories draw from various sources in Eastern philosophy, Theosophy and traditional religions, including shamanism, Native American spirituality and Wicca.[28] Although this energy is claimed to be impersonal and nonreligious, in practice it frequently takes on personality so that healing modalities become a "channeling" or manipulation of spirits.

From a scientific perspective, proponents of energy-based theories vacillate between two extremes. Some advocates dismiss science entirely and claim the effectiveness of the associated modalities through anecdotal evidence. Others have attempted to use both quantitative and qualitative research methods to prove they work. Results, however, remain inconclusive.[29] Some have attempted to blend modern physics with Eastern mysticism[30] but have made quantum leaps in logic and reality in the process.[31]

Pagan Religion Revived

Some nurses—theorists, educators and practitioners—are affirming pagan religions as a source of new creativity and power. The natural world of pagan religion, like that of traditional religions, is alive. "Not only humans, but also animals, plants, and even rocks, sand, and water are thought to have personalities, wills, and life forces."[32] Most Western advocates of these religions hold a romantic view of them, seeing them as bringing mystery and harmony into human life. What they fail to understand is that in these worlds people are at the mercy of capricious invisible ancestors, demons, witches, ghosts, heavenly bodies, local gods and impersonal forces of good and evil.

In the pagan worldview a supreme god is distant and unconcerned about the daily problems of life: sickness, death, bad luck and accidents. The only defense for humans is to gain power over these capricious spirits and forces that cause their problems. "Power, not truth, is the central human concern in this worldview."[33]

Today, accounts of fertility rites, white witchcraft, divination, palmistry, fortune-telling and astrology are gaining credibility and acceptance. Many bookstores have large sections devoted to Wicca and the occult. Tabloids carry stories of ghosts, witchcraft, evil-eye curses and fulfilled prophecies. Nurse researcher Sharon Fish has documented the close ties between some of the energy therapies being advocated by nurses who call themselves healers and Theosophy, an admittedly occult philosophy.[34]

Such beliefs, suppressed during the reign of science, have never fully left the Western mind. Below the level of orthodox Christianity an assortment of folk religious beliefs persisted, handed down by word of mouth, despite the opposition of church leaders and the ridicule of scientists.[35] At the center of these folk religions are the shaman and the practice of magic. Historian of religion Mircea Eliade characterizes the shaman as one who communicates with the spirits in an ecstatic trance. He or she performs miraculous cures and predicts future events. Shamans serve as mediators between ordinary people and the spirit world.[36]

Shamanism is gaining credibility in nursing today.[37] Some nurses even refer to themselves as shamans. The healer in energy-based therapies like therapeutic touch fills the role of the shaman when manipulating and directing "life energy" by hand and body movements, mental concentration or both.[38] Even the Christian practice of praying for the sick is sometimes interpreted in the language of shamanism.[39]

Shamanism is associated with magic, the attempt to influence people and events by supernatural or occult means. Black magic attempts to produce evil results through such methods as curses, spells, destruction of models of one's enemy and alliance with evil spirits. White magic tries to undo curses and spells, and to use occult forces for the good of oneself and others.[40] The magician tries to compel a spirit to work for him or her or follows a pattern of occult practices to bend psychic forces to do the magician's will. Magic is carried out by specific rituals and methods known only to those who are initiates into the practice. Healers who practice these rituals often refer to themselves as white witches.[41]

So far in this chapter we have presented the worldviews that have shaped and are shaping nursing theory—the modern worldview and the postmodern worldview. We agree that theories of nursing based on the modern mechanistic worldview are not adequate to undergird the practice of nursing. Theories that reduce persons by materialistic explanations and ignore the spiritual realm can never satisfactorily encompass the richness of nursing: caring for people in life and death, in times of high joy and crushing sorrow.

However, we challenge the idea that theories based on pagan religions are the answer. Returning to shamanism and spiritism where we must appease spirits, or to magic where we seek to dominate reality for our own ends through rituals and formulas, will lead to dehumanization, disillusionment and spiritual oppression. The worldviews undergirding the practices and ways of thinking that face Sonja, Maria and Karen promise much but offer only illusions. Instead, we believe that nurses need to re-examine the view of reality portrayed in the Bible. We turn to that worldview in the next chapter.

3

A Biblical
Worldview
for Nursing

THE BEGINNINGS OF ORGANIZED NURSING IN NORWAY ILLUS-
trate a common pattern for how nursing became established around the
world. Ingeborg Gjersvik tells the story:

> Around 1850 Norway experienced a spiritual awakening which mo-
> tivated an important social awakening. People began to see the need
> to care for the sick and the poor. The very thought of women caring
> for sick people outside of their own families, and furthermore estab-
> lishing a training course to do so, was unheard of and unacceptable in
> Norwegian society at that time. However, many prayer groups were
> formed, asking for God's guidance in this matter.[1]

The answer to their prayers came through Cathinka Guldberg, a pastor's
daughter who used to make home visits to the sick with her father. One
night Cathinka discovered that a homeless woman, who had been going
from door to door begging for shelter, had been found frozen to death in
the snow. Deeply convicted, Cathinka prayed about how she could make a
difference. Soon afterwards, she found a leaflet about the Kaiserswerth
Deaconess community and considered it an answer to her prayers. She
studied nursing in Kaiserswerth, then returned to begin a nurses' training

program for deaconesses. The school expanded to include lay nurses. Then additional nursing schools were established, and nursing spread throughout Norway.

As nursing history demonstrates over and over, something radically different has happened in society through the Christian church. Second-century theologian Tertullian noted:

> It is our care of the helpless, our practice of loving kindness that brands us in the eyes of many of our opponents. "Only look," they say, "how they love one another! Look how they are prepared to die for one another."[2]

During a devastating third-century plague, historian Eusebius of Caesarea recorded:

> The Christians were the only people who amid such terrible ills, showed their fellow-feelings and humanity by their actions. Day by day some would busy themselves by attending to the dead and burying them; others gathered in one spot all who were afflicted by hunger throughout the whole city and give them bread.[3]

Nursing grew out of a Christian worldview, in response to Jesus' teaching and example of caring for the sick. What was it about the Christian worldview that motivated the early church to reach out to the poor, the sick and the marginalized?

While other worldviews of the time focused on gaining control of the physical elements and spiritual powers, the early Christians looked instead to God as one who deserved love and obedience and who inspired loving service to others. As we have seen, that tradition of caring for others in the form of nursing has continued throughout church history.

What we believe about God shapes our understanding of human persons and the environment in which we find ourselves. That, in turn, informs our concept of health and directs us to the means by which we nurture one another toward health and healing (see figure 1). So as Christians we begin with a *theology* of nursing, more than a philosophy or theory. If we truly believe what we say we believe about God, we cannot help but act in obedience to him, which means communicating the good news of salvation, health and healing through word and deed.

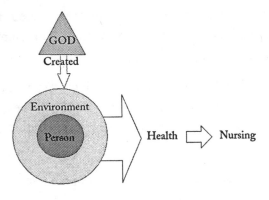

Figure 1. Nursing from a Christian perspective

The Christian worldview is neither the mechanistic understanding of modernism nor the impersonal energy field of the New Paradigm (postmodernism) but is characterized by personal relationship with God and other people.

The Christian worldview affirms good empirical science and the appropriate use of technology. They are gifts from God to be used for the benefit of creation. The methods of science give us knowledge of the physical aspects of creation. However, science has its limits. The personal, spiritual aspects of creation are veiled, and, while manifested in the physical world, they cannot be explained by science. The meaning of the personal and spiritual are seen only in the context of a larger worldview.

Christians also affirm many of the concerns and goals of the New Paradigm, although our understanding of the concepts involved may differ. We share the concern for a more personal approach to health care, including the use of touch. We hold a holistic view of the person and recognize the need to provide comfort in human suffering. The Christian worldview includes the reality of the spiritual and unseen and the importance of faith and prayer. We recognize that there may be forms of physical energy that we cannot yet measure, and we reject the scientism that reduces all reality to physical or material phenomena.

The uniqueness of Christ-inspired nursing lies in its emphasis on caring for the whole person as embodied, respecting each person as created in the image of God. It is both a science and an art, but primarily it is a response to God's grace and a reflection of his character.

Christian Uniqueness

While Christian values such as unconditional love and compassionate caring have been widely appreciated, even by postmodern nurses, other aspects of Christian faith are coming under intense criticism. Consider the following discussion we recently had with a group of nursing faculty members.

"With increased diversity and the rapid proliferation of other religions in our society, nursing has to become more inclusive," one professor explained, then continued, "we have to be more open-minded and approach spirituality from a broader perspective."

Another added, "It is presumptuous for Christians to think they can know God better than people of other religions do. Although the Christian faith is right for me, I think we have to respect their traditions as well."

"All truth is God's truth," interjected another. "If alternative therapies work, we should use them, regardless of the worldview behind them."

While all of these nurses were Christians, they were also postmodern in their understanding of spirituality. Their comments echoed the spirit of our age.

A Christian worldview cannot simply be superimposed on any other worldview. One of the unique features of Christianity—the one that grates most on the postmodern conscience—is *the scandal of particularity*. The Bible teaches that God singled out one people (the Hebrews) at a particular time and place in history to whom to reveal himself as the only true God. He drew firm boundaries, requiring absolute faithfulness. Any worship of other gods he labeled idolatry or spiritual adultery. He then took on human flesh in the one person of Jesus Christ, who said, "I am the way, and the truth, and the life. No one comes to the Father except through me" (Jn 14:6). You can't get much more exclusive. However, Jesus also said:

> I am the bread of life. Whoever comes to me will never be hungry, and whoever believes in me will never be thirsty. . . . This is indeed the will of my Father, that all who see the Son and believe in him may have eternal life; and I will raise them up on the last day. (Jn 6:35, 40)

God's offer of salvation is, in reality, the most *inclusive* belief system. He calls all of creation into relationship with himself. It is a free gift, but it is on his terms. When Job, in the Old Testament, questioned God's design, the Lord responded by charging, "Where were you when I laid the foundation of the earth? Tell me, if you have understanding" (Job 38:4). When we presume to know a better way than what God has revealed to us in Scripture, we are like children crying, "Everybody else is doing it!" Every wise parent knows that what "everybody else" is doing is not necessarily right or good. The call to be spiritually inclusive falsely masquerades as virtue, when in truth it is simply rebellion against God. Furthermore, the kind of tolerance advocated by many people in our society is merely indifference, not kindness and compassion.

God in the Bible

A theology of nursing must be centered in Christian doctrine as contained in the Scriptures and affirmed by the historic Christian creeds. Although some Christian traditions would like to avoid referring to creedal formulations, preferring instead to claim "Christ alone" as their only creed, in today's religious climate the terms *God, Jesus* and *Christ* mean many different things. The historic creeds of the church provide a definitive summary of essential theological understandings. Theologian Timothy Lull explains:

> The early church discovered it could not live by Scripture alone in the simple sense of settling every question on the basis of biblical teaching. Some rule of faith was needed to distinguish true Christians from those many others who used Christian writings—and even the person

of Jesus Christ—as a character in a very different story. The ancient world was full of competing religious groups, almost any one of which could incorporate the Jesus story in some way and use him for their own purposes.

The three Creeds specify the precise Jesus story which is the authentic witness of the Bible. They speak with increasing precision and length about the God who loved the world and about his coming among us in Jesus Christ. They speak of one God who made the world, but did not stand afar off when human beings fell into sin. Rather, "for us and for our salvation he came down from heaven and . . . was made man."[4]

The three creeds Lull references are the Apostles', Nicene and Athanasian Creeds. The Apostles' Creed was developed in the second century out of a baptismal liturgy used by the church in Rome. The Nicene Creed was constructed by the Council of Nicea in 325 and revised to its present form in 381, to counter the heresy of Arianism (which denied the divinity of Christ). The Athanasian Creed developed in about the fifth century.

The trinitarian nature of God—Father, Son and Holy Spirit—forms the basic structure for each of the historic creeds. God is described as Creator of the universe, who established both time and eternity; Redeemer of the world, who entered history in human form to suffer and die for our sins; and Sanctifier of his people, who continues to dwell among and within us. We can know God personally, but we cannot become God or force him to do our bidding. Furthermore, we can know God only as he reveals himself to us. We cannot merely shape God into whatever we want him to be. The Bible calls that *idolatry*.[5]

God requires our obedience and faithfulness, and he cannot be manipulated or controlled (Job 38:4—40:1; Is 43:13). He is both transcendent (beyond us) and immanent (with us). The prophet Isaiah tells us:

For thus says the high and lofty one who inhabits eternity, whose name is Holy: I dwell in the high and holy place, and also with those who are contrite and humble in spirit, to revive the spirit of the humble, and to revive the heart of the contrite. (Is 57:15)

We are to worship God in spirit and in truth (Jn 4:23), not turn to him as a good luck charm or try to bargain with him. He is not a celestial candy machine, ready to churn out treats if we insert the right coins.

Just as the Christian creeds were developed in times of upheaval and controversy, when many conflicting views of God vied for adherents in the church, we need to clearly identify the essential components of Christian theology today. The problem of heterodoxy is not new. Many old heresies simply reappear in new forms, but as our culture moves from modernism to postmodernism, the lines may once again need to be drawn in new places. Jesus warned that false doctrines would develop and that his followers would need discernment:

> Not everyone who says to me, "Lord, Lord," will enter the kingdom of heaven, but only the one who does the will of my Father in heaven. On that day many will say to me, "Lord, Lord, did we not prophesy in your name, and cast out demons in your name, and do many deeds of power in your name?" Then I will declare to them, "I never knew you; go away from me, you evildoers." (Mt 7:21-23)

At strategic points in history ecclesiastical councils, reformations and revivals developed to root out heresy and reform the church. The reformers knew that the way people viewed God not only affected their worship and personal salvation but also shaped their ethics and morality—the way they related to one another, and their use and abuse of power. We can see these results in church history as it relates to nursing history. With a few exceptions, during times when the church remained faithful to Scripture and orthodox in beliefs, nursing flourished. When the church grew weak and corrupt, nursing suffered and declined.[6]

To see the effects of our belief systems on nursing practice today, we will first look at what we know about God, then briefly compare the concepts of the nursing metaparadigm in the biblical worldview to the two other worldviews that prevail in our culture today, modernism and postmodernism (New Paradigm). The chapters that follow will further explore the practical implications of the biblical worldview and other worldviews in the nursing metaparadigm. In the process we will discover some of the reasons why the present health care system has evolved into the impersonal, highly technological "body shop" approach of managed care, while at the same time it has turned to energy-based theories with their widening array of often bizarre and unproven alternative therapies. We aim to propose a more satisfying alternative.

God the Creator

When St. Paul preached to Greek philosophers in Athens, he commended them for being very religious and even erecting an altar to an unknown god. He claimed to know who this god was: "The God who made the world and everything in it, he who is the Lord of heaven and of earth . . . he himself gives to all mortals life and breath and all things. From one ancestor he made all nations to inhabit the whole earth . . . he is not far from each of us" (Acts 17:22-27). Paul then quoted two of their poets, "For 'In him [God] we live and move and have our being'; as even some of your own poets have said, 'For we too are his offspring' " (Acts 17:28). Paul was asserting what Jews and Christians believe, that God alone is the only uncreated reality, the only being who is eternally self-existent. All else that exists, living and nonliving, is created and sustained by the Creator.

We are God's offspring in the sense that he created us. By asserting that all humanity descended from one ancestor, Paul affirmed the unity of the human race as well as the source of our life in God. Some of the Athenians believed that their race had sprung from the soil of their city. Paul did not mean that humans were a mere manifestation of a universal divinity in which they would someday lose their individual existence. What he did mean was that we are totally dependent upon God for our life, *even if we do not recognize it.*[7]

While all created things are dependent upon the Creator, God, on the other hand, has life in himself. He is self-existent. Jesus said, "For just as the Father has life in himself, so he has granted the Son also to have life in himself" (Jn 5:26). Jesus, the Son, was both God and human (a mystery indeed), and here he was claiming to have the same self-existent life as God the Father. He spoke these words in the context of teaching about the resurrection of all who have ever lived and died. St. Paul wrote of Jesus Christ:

He is the image of the invisible God, the firstborn of all creation; for in him all things in heaven and on earth were created, things visible and invisible, whether thrones or dominions or rulers or powers—all things have been created through him and for him. He himself is before all things, and in him all things hold together (Col 1:15-17).

A Loving Heavenly Father

Our knowledge of God is not something we can use to gain power over others. If we try it, we risk God's rejection (see the quote from Mt 7 above). Knowing God doesn't convey social status; instead, it gives us a family identity. We understand God in terms of relationship—a relationship of faithfulness and trust. The Bible provides several vivid analogies. We relate to God as a child to a parent, as a bride to her husband, and as a branch to the vine. These are intimate and essential relationships, necessary to create, sustain and nurture life itself.

We understand God as Creator most clearly when we see him as our loving heavenly Father. While many people struggle with the idea of God as Father because their relationship with an earthly father was marred, that does not negate the imagery. For it is in looking at God that we see how a father *should* relate to his children. Martin Luther, in constructing his *Small Catechism,* an instructional guide for children, put it this way:

I believe that God has created me together with all creatures. God has given me and still preserves my body and soul: eyes, ears, and all limbs and senses; reason and mental faculties. In addition, God daily and abundantly provides shoes and clothing, food and drink, house and home, spouse and clothing, fields, livestock, and all property—along with all the necessities and nourishment for this body and life. God protects me against all danger and shields and preserves me from all evil. God does all this out of pure, fatherly, and divine goodness and mercy, without any merit or worthiness of mine at all! For this I owe it to God to thank and praise, serve and obey him. This is most certainly true.[8]

We can learn a great deal about God from parenthood. In many ways we are all like two-year-olds who have broken away from our parents in a toy store. Surrounded by delightful playthings, we assume that they have been put there for us. We do not realize that they belong to someone else and will cost our parents dearly if we break them. Neither do we see the dangers that surround us. We cannot read the labels that say "Not Safe for Children Under Three." Nor do we realize that kidnappers may be lurking in the aisles waiting to abduct children. Furthermore, it does not occur to us that our parents may be frantically looking for us, while we wander gleefully among the goodies.

Being the mother of teenagers has given me (Judy) even more insights into God's relationship with his people who are constantly trying to establish independence from him. It is a terribly personal and protective role. You watch your son go out, boldly naive to the dangers that await him—but you let him go, knowing that he must learn from the "school of hard knocks." You deny your daughter many of her deep desires, even when you could probably afford to buy them and would love to lavish them upon her, because you realize that doing so would only produce an arrogant, selfish child. You trust your good name to your children, only to receive a detention slip in the mail because one of them has called the teacher an inappropriate name. It is hard to be a parent, and yet we continue to love and nurture our children regardless of their behavior, to stick by them and to discipline them. Most of the time they don't understand or appreciate what we do—the carefully prepared meal is left uneaten, the intended surprise gift of clothing is left in a heap and never worn, the rules are broken. You become invisible and unacknowledged when their friends are present. I'm beginning to understand how God's heart is grieved by our unfaithfulness.

But the love and pain we feel as parents is nothing compared to the great love our heavenly Father has for us. Jesus tells us, "If you then, who are evil, know how to give good gifts to your children, how much more will your Father in heaven give good things to those who ask him!" (Mt 7:11). God faces the same tensions in his relationship to us, yet he remains absolutely faithful. The psalmist tells us, "As a father has compassion for his children, so the LORD has compassion for those who fear him" (Ps 103:13). The prophet Hosea quotes God as saying:

When Israel was a child, I loved him,
    and out of Egypt I called my son.
The more I called them,
    the more they went from me;
they kept sacrificing to the Baals,
    and offering incense to idols.
Yet it was I who taught Ephraim to walk,
    I took them up in my arms;
    but they did not know that I healed them.
I led them with cords of human kindness,
    with bands of love.
I was to them like those
    who lift infants to their cheeks.
    I bent down to them and fed them. (Hos 11:1-4)

The fact that God is our Creator and Father indicates that we owe him our full allegiance and gratitude. Although we represent him in all that we do, we can never impersonate him, much less become God. However, the relationship we experience with God is intended to be one of joy and delight. The *Westminster Shorter Catechism* puts it beautifully:

Q1: What is the chief end of man?

A1: Man's chief end is to glorify God, and to enjoy him forever.

The implications of this fatherly relationship with God for nursing are abundant. We serve a loving God who truly cares for us—and for our patients. He is concerned about our nutrition, hydration and appearance (Mt 6:25-34). He knows us intimately, even the number of hairs on our heads (Mt 10:30); he calls us by name (Is 43:1). Not only is he aware of human suffering, he walks with us through it (Ex 3:12; Is 43:2) and suffers with us (Heb 2:9). We can trust him in the midst of our suffering, just as young children trust their parents, because we know he is faithful. First Peter 4:19 tells us, "Therefore, let those suffering in accordance with God's will entrust themselves to a faithful Creator, while continuing to do good."

While the biblical understanding of God certainly does not answer all the *why?* questions, it puts them into perspective. Our children don't understand why they have to eat their vegetables, or struggle through learning multiplication tables, or suffer the pain of immunizations, but as parents we know what is best for them. In the same way, we do not know why our patients suffer and die, but we can be assured that God loves them and cares for them far more than we do. What a contrast to the modernist worldview that sees God (if he exists at all) as dispassionate and uninvolved with creation. The contrast is even starker when compared to the view of God as impersonal energy served by an array of amoral spirits who must be manipulated and appeased.

God in Human Form

God's relationship to his people is most clearly demonstrated in Jesus Christ. Jesus is not just a good example or cosmic consciousness. He is Almighty God himself who came to live among us as fully human. He shared our struggles, experienced pain, suffered, and died so that we could be restored to full relationship with God, our heavenly Father.

> Since, then, we have a great high priest who has passed through the heavens, Jesus, the Son of God, let us hold fast to our confession. For we do not have a high priest who is unable to sympathize with our weaknesses, but we have one who in every respect has been tested as we are, yet without sin. Let us therefore approach the throne of grace with boldness, so that we may receive mercy and find grace to help in time of need. (Heb 4:14-16)

In Jesus we see God's presence with us in concrete terms. We know God is concerned about human illness and suffering because we can read about how Jesus healed the sick, cast out demons and even raised the dead. Furthermore, his whole earthly life was ordered around the ultimate purpose of going to the cross to suffer *for* us so that we could escape suffering. First Peter 2:24 tells us, "He himself bore our sins in his body on the cross, so that, free from sins, we might live for righteousness; by his wounds you have been healed."

It is through Jesus that we receive the motivation and power to care for others. He is the clear demonstration of God's love for us (Jn 3:16; 1 Jn 3:1), and it is because he first loved us that we can love others (1 Jn 4:19).

Furthermore, he has blessed and commissioned us to go out in his name, continuing his works of caring, healing and exorcism (Mt 28:19-20; Mk 16:17; Lk 10:9). In John 14:12 Jesus tells us, "The one who believes in me will also do the works that I do and, in fact, will do greater works than these."

Spirit of the Living God

We experience God's ongoing intimate involvement in our lives through the work of the Holy Spirit. The Holy Spirit is not an energy field we can transmit, our own spark of divinity, or God's female alter ego, but the awesome otherness of God who chooses to dwell in our hearts and work in our midst. Soon before his death, Jesus said that he would send the Holy Spirit as Counselor (Advocate) to be with us forever (Jn 14:16). This Spirit teaches us all things and guides us into truth. He comes from God the Father and bears witness to Jesus (Jn 14:25; 15:26; 16:13). The apostle Paul tells us:

> Likewise the Spirit helps us in our weakness; for we do not know how to pray as we ought, but that very Spirit intercedes with sighs too deep for words. And God, who searches the heart, knows what is the mind of the Spirit, because the Spirit intercedes for the saints according to the will of God. (Rom 8:26-27)

The Holy Spirit bestows gifts upon us and produces godly fruit in our lives. The *gifts* are those things that empower us to serve others in Christ's name—wisdom, knowledge, faith, service, giving aid, acts of mercy, healing, working miracles, teaching, prophecy, exhortation, discernment of spirits, and tongues (Rom 12:6-8; 1 Cor 12:8-10). Through these gifts we are able to participate in the work of God's kingdom. We are not left on our own to try to conjure up the power and ability to face the weight of suffering and death in nursing; the Holy Spirit gives us all that we need. Once we realize that we do all good things in partnership with God, we can relax and allow him to work through us. Life—including nursing—becomes an amazing adventure where we are constantly surprised by God's great goodness.

The *fruit* of the Spirit is the character of God demonstrated in our lives—love, joy, peace, patience, kindness, generosity, faithfulness, gentleness and self-control (Gal 5:22-23). Again, these are not personal accomplishments we have to strive toward. They are the natural results of having the Holy Spirit living within us. Jesus said, "I am the vine, you are the branches. Those who abide in me and I in them bear much fruit, because apart from me you can do nothing" (Jn 15:5). As we spend time with God in prayer and live our lives in obedience to him, we will demonstrate the fruit of his Spirit and experience his power in our daily lives—while at the same time becoming intensely aware of our own inadequacy and sinfulness.

The only appropriate response to an encounter with this true God is a humble recognition of our own sinfulness and powerlessness. John tells us that the Holy Spirit will "prove the world wrong about sin and righteousness and judgment" (Jn 16:8). When we stand before our Holy God, we lose any of our culture's pretensions about being "basically good" or having "a basically positive direction."[9] The prophet Isaiah vividly described his response to an awesome encounter with God:

> And I said: "Woe is me! I am lost, for I am a man of unclean lips, and
> I live among a people of unclean lips; yet my eyes have seen the King,
> the LORD of hosts!" (Is 6:5)

Our culture tends to view this recognition of human sinfulness as negative and goes to great lengths to avoid it. However, the biblical understanding of sin is one of the most liberating theological concepts in Christian doctrine. How else can we explain the ravages of war, illness, accidents, natural disasters and all the abuse and violence in human relationships? Even those who do not acknowledge God insist that we must recognize our problems before we can do anything about them. It is our confession of sin that drives us to Jesus Christ as Savior to find forgiveness and redemption. It restores our perspective to see that God is on his throne, his kingdom is secure. Confessing our own sinfulness and experiencing God's forgiveness frees us to delight in the joy of his salvation. This relationship of grace overflows into praise to God and a life of service to humanity. Nursing, as a public ministry of the church, developed out of this understanding of sin and redemption.

The Seen and Unseen

The biblical worldview includes a spiritual dimension—things that we cannot see. In our own culture, scientism has blinded us to the reality of the spiritual world. The Bible affirms that the personal, spiritual, unseen world is real and was created by God (Eph 6:12). The Nicene Creed affirms: "We believe in one God, the Father, the Almighty, maker of heaven and earth, of all that is, seen and unseen."

Spiritual beings are not merely psychological projections. They are personal, intelligent beings, and they have intentions toward us (Lk 22:31; 1 Pet 5:8-9; Jas 4:7). One form of spiritual beings, angels, are God's servants under his authority (Col 1:16; Heb 1:14). God often directs them to protect and shelter his people (Gen 19:15; 1 Kings 19:5-7; Mt 4:6; Lk 1:30; 4:10; 22:43).

Another form of spiritual beings, evil spirits or demons, were also created by God but rebelled against him. They are beings who intend to deceive us about God and to control us, ultimately destroying us. We are not to worship angels or evil spirits or enter into collusion with them (Ps 91:11; Mt 26:53; Lk 4:10; Col 2:18).

Because demons deceive and destroy, and because they are spiritually powerful and crafty, we are to have no dealings with them (1 Cor 10:20-21; 2 Cor 2:11; 1 Tim 4:1). Christians are protected from demons' power by being in Christ Jesus, but they constantly tempt us (Mt 28:18; Jn 8:31-32; Acts 19:11-20; Eph 6:11). God has opened the *only* legitimate way for spiritual life—through Jesus Christ (Mt 11:27; Jn 14:6).

As we have noted already, the four basic concepts that shape the nature of nursing are the *person*, the *environment*, *health* and *nursing*. We have found it necessary to begin with the concept of God to make sense of the concepts that follow. In the remainder of this chapter we will provide some basic definitions and understandings based on a Christian worldview. They are summarized in figure 2, "Worldviews in Brief." Each concept will be more fully explored in the following chapters.

Person

Fawcett describes the person as "the recipient of nursing, including individuals, families, communities, and other groups."[10] We would also include the nurse as a person, as well as all those human beings who are *not* presently recipients of nursing care.

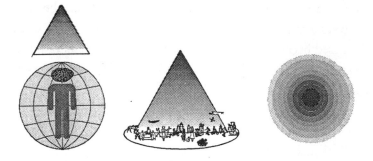

Concept	Modern	Biblical	Postmodern
God	Transcendent, acknowledged but not involved in daily life, Unmoved Prime Mover	Immanent *and* transcendent, personal, triune: Creator, Redeemer, Sanctifier, Sovereign Lord of the Universe	Immanent, impersonal, One (with all things), Energy *(chi, ki, prana, life force)*
Truth	Objective—reason, empirical science	Both objective (science) and subjective (experience); must be tested by Scripture. Ultimately it is Jesus Christ.	Subjective—relative, experiential, personally constructed
Environment	Physical matter	All of creation, physical and spiritual, created good but polluted by sin, distinct from God but under his control	Spiritual energy with no distinctions, only graded intensities, Gaia
Person	Body/soul dualism, autonomous	Created in image of God, sinful, integrated, relational (to God and others)	Energy field, body illusory, divine, related by collective unconscious
Health	Absence of disease	*Shalom*	Expanded consciousness
Nursing	Conquering illness through technology and scientifically determined care, medical model	Compassionate care for whole person to foster *shalom*, comfort for suffering and dying, response to God's love	Holistic, but caring is increasingly in the mind, moving away from caring for the body; New Paradigm
Spiritual Care	Respect for individual's religious preference	Fostering relationship with God, communicating gospel in word and deed	Comfort through technique and ritual, alternative therapies

Figure 2. Worldviews in brief

In Western dualism the person is reduced to what can be seen—anatomy and physiology. Although there is some recognition of the mind, or soul, it is dismissed because it cannot be quantified and measured. Health care in this worldview is medical and surgical technology. In the New Paradigm the person is merely "congealed energy." Health care involves manipulating the energy, or vital life force, to restore balance. Increasingly, it is openly moving toward manipulation of spirits as well.

Biblical theism views all people as created by God in his image (Gen 1:26) to live in loving relationship with God, self and others (Deut 6:4-6; Mt 22:37-39) and to be responsible stewards of the environment (Gen 1:26). Every person is separated from God by sin, but that relationship is restored by grace through faith in Jesus Christ, in whom we are redeemed and sanctified by the Holy Spirit (Rom 3:22-28; 1 Cor 6:11). The person is a physically, psychosocially and spiritually integrated being with intrinsic value and significance (Ps 8:4-8; 1 Thess 5:23; Heb 2:11-17). Each person is responsible to live a healthful lifestyle (1 Cor 3:16-17; Eph 5:29) and to promote health (Ex 15:26; 3 Jn 2), but also to find meaning in suffering and death (Rom 5:3-5; 1 Cor 15:54; 1 Thess 4:13-14).

Environment

According to Fawcett the *environment* "refers to the person's significant others and physical surroundings, as well as to the setting in which nursing occurs, which ranges from the person's home to clinical agencies to society as a whole."[11]

How do worldviews affect the context of nursing? Look around you. If you are in a high-tech, low-touch setting, your environment has probably been shaped by Western dualism. If you are surrounded by colleagues practicing therapeutic touch and crystal therapy, you have entered the New Paradigm. If you are a parish nurse in a church, your practice is probably informed by Christian theology. None of these settings will be purely one worldview; in fact, several worldviews may be operating in tension, but usually one of the three predominates and will eventually win out.

Human relationships—the significant others in the environment—will also differ according to a person's worldview. Western dualism tends toward utilitarianism. Human value is determined by whatever seems best for society and, on a personal level, whatever is most beneficial to me. Despite its appeal to be more caring and holistic, the New Paradigm tends to ultimately discount personal relationship entirely. If people are merely energy fields, they are already related (in an impersonal way) to one another and everything else in the world; there are no distinctions, only graded intensities. However, in biblical theism we find human community and practical caring at the deepest level.

The physical environment is receiving a great deal of attention today. Scientists wrestle with the problem of global warming, using advanced technology and quantitative research. Ecofeminists turn to becoming one with nature and conduct services worshiping "Earth Mother." Christians are also trying to determine appropriate ways to be good stewards of creation, caring for the earth in responsible ways. The various worldviews, however, approach the environment from widely different perspectives. Some are compatible with biblical theism, and some are clearly incompatible.

According to the Bible the world was created by God, who declared it *good* (Gen 1). The environment has been polluted by sin and awaits redemption by God (Rom 8:22). The environment includes both physical and spiritual realities (Col 1:16) and encompasses the human community (Ps 24:1) and culture. The creation is separate from God (Is 55:8-9). It is not God and cannot become God (Gen 2:7; Ex 20:23; Is 44:6-20). Each person has the responsibility to care for the environment as a steward of God's gifts (Gen 1:28; 1 Pet 4:10). The environment can bring both healing and illness. The effects of pollution and stress can contribute to disease. A clean, supportive environment can bring refreshment and healing. Because the environment affects human health, nurses have the responsibility to care for and improve the environment.

Health

Health is the goal of nursing, but definitions of health vary greatly in our society and from culture to culture. The way we define health will have major ramifications in the way we practice nursing. It will shape our assessments and interventions, as well as the way we determine success.

For the Western dualist health is simply the absence of disease. The goal of nursing is to maintain optimal biological functioning, often with little regard for emotional and spiritual concerns. The extreme application of this definition has led to abuses of heroic measures, such as repeatedly resuscitating terminally ill cancer patients or maintaining brain-dead persons on life-support systems. However, we also see it reflected in nursing's attempts to quantify the causes and effects in nursing practice: nursing process, nursing diagnosis and classifying interventions and outcomes. We can appreciate many of the positive results in patient care gained through viewing health as the absence of disease, but its usefulness is limited. Not all people respond to prescribed policies and procedures, or drugs and treatments, in the same way. Dualism does not account for the spiritual and unseen—the *human factor.*

The New Paradigm attempts to deal with the human factor and take into account the emotional and spiritual variables that make each individual unique. In the New Paradigm, health is seen as something that you must define for yourself. Margaret Newman sees health as "expanding consciousness."[12] Rosemarie Parse sees it as "the quality of life as experienced by the person."[13] The problem with these definitions of health is that nursing ends up with no goals, or at best conflicting goals. Nursing may range from standing by without any physical interventions to performing potentially harmful procedures that the patient desires. The movement toward assisted suicide grows out of this loose definition of health.

In biblical theism wellness, or health, is being able to live as God created us to be—as an integrated whole living in loving relationship with God, self and others (Ps 16). It is dependent on the cross and resurrection of Jesus Christ (Is 53:5; 1 Pet 2:24). Health is central to the Old Testament concept of *shalom* (Ps 38:3; Jer 33:6) and the New Testament understanding of *salvation* (Lk 18:42). The presence of sin in the world and the predilection of each person to sin impinge on health spiritually, physically and psychosocially (Ex 20:5; Ps 32:3-4; Lk 5:17-25). Physical or psychosocial dysfunction can also cause spiritual distress (Job 16:7-9; Ps 13; 22). While God's ultimate plan for us is complete health, a person can be spiritually healthy while physically or psychosocially limited (1 Cor 1:27-29; 2 Cor 11:7-9). Health is the goal of nursing and a sign of the kingdom of God (Rev 21:1-7).

Nursing

We have already discussed how shifting worldviews have brought tremendous changes to nursing and health care. In later chapters we will examine the roots and implications of these paradigm shifts, but here we want to clearly establish what we are talking about as *nursing*. In biblical theism, nursing is a ministry of compassionate care for the whole person, in response to God's grace, which aims to foster optimum health *(shalom)* and bring comfort in suffering and death. Nursing includes the comprehensive physical, psychosocial and spiritual care of individuals in the context of families and communities. Because the healing work of Christ is a sign of the kingdom and a response to God's mercy (Lk 10:1-9), nurses follow Christ's command to "go and do likewise" (Lk 10:37). Nurses compassionately care for anyone in need, regardless of ethnic identity, race, gender, age, status, diagnosis or ability to pay (Is 61:1-3; Mt 25:35-36; Lk 4:18-19; 16:19-25; Gal 3:28).

The actual tasks of nursing may vary as needs, contexts and resources change, but Christian nursing is always a faithful response to God's gift of salvation. We love others because God first loved us. That love is lived out in compassionate action toward our neighbors.

Part Two

The Person as the Focus of Nursing

4

What Does It Mean
to Be Human?

THE ATMOSPHERE IN THE NEWBORN NURSERY SEEMED strangely tense when Alice reported for work on Monday morning. A tightly-wrapped bundle in a far corner had ignited the controversy. Born during the night shift, Baby Morgan appeared healthy and beautiful at first glance, but the stocking cap covered an anencephalic head. The pediatrician raged that the baby should have been aborted early in the pregnancy. After all, a scan had revealed the problem months ago. The parents knew the diagnosis but chose to carry the baby to term anyway. Dr. Mabry left a verbal "do not feed, do not treat" order and stomped out.

After the physician left, Alice gently lifted Baby Morgan out of his crib and held him close. His high-pitched wailing stopped and his tiny body relaxed. Alice looked at his perfectly formed face and thought of the joy she had felt when her own children were born. She knew she would not be able to honor the physician's order. Deep in her being she realized that this child, imperfect though he might be, was created in the image of God.

The Image of God
The Christian understanding of human beings as created in the image of

God bestows dignity and honor on every person, regardless of social, mental or physical status. It forms the basis of Western society's understanding of human rights and undergirds our legal system as well as our health care and social service agencies. But challenges from both modernism and postmodernism threaten to change this basic assumption.

Consider this introductory statement in a textbook on family systems theory:

> [Bowen] believed that a major obstacle to the acceptance of human behavior as a proper subject for scientific inquiry is that, traditionally, humankind has tended to consider itself a unique form of life, one with a special place in God's plan. Such self-glorification precludes our seeing the myriad ways we act just like other forms of life.[1]

The postmodern argument with viewing persons as the image of God (*imago Dei*) takes a different tack. Drawing from an eclectic array of ancient and newly constructed religions and philosophies, as we have seen, many are beginning to view the earth as a living organism. Kleffel explains, "Humans are one functioning part of the totality and act in harmony within the organism."[2] In other words, human life is no more valuable than a rock or a raccoon. The philosophy reveals itself in the tee-shirt slogan borne by Margie, a junior student: "Save the rats, experiment on people."

Recognizing the *imago Dei* in each human being does suggest that we have a special place in God's plan, with serious moral consequences. We can own dogs, cats and cattle, but not human slaves. We eat chickens and pigs for dinner, but not people—even our enemies. We shoot lame horses, but not disabled veterans. It was the *imago Dei* that drove Mother Teresa to care for the sick and dying in Calcutta, as it has motivated Christians throughout the centuries to care for the poor, the sick and the disenfranchised. Whenever a society has ceased to recognize the image of God in human beings, whether in the name of science, political ideology, religion or simply greed, serious moral decay soon followed. We have only to look at the Nazi Holocaust, the decline of compassionate health care under the Communist regimes and our own profit-driven health care system for vivid illustrations.

What is the *imago Dei*? The concept begins in Genesis 1:26:

Then God said, "Let us make humankind in our image, according to our likeness; and let them have dominion over the fish of the sea, and over the birds of the air, and over the cattle, and over all the wild animals of the earth, and over every creeping thing that creeps upon the earth."

This single verse delivers a powerful threefold message. First, we are created by a personal God who designed us for a relationship with himself. Second, we somehow reflect the nature of this God. And finally, God gives us a position of responsibility and authority over the rest of creation.

To be created in the image of God means that we must look to God for our meaning, purpose and direction. It also makes us thinking, feeling, willing, relational creatures who reflect these attributes of our Creator. In order to understand ourselves in any depth, we must first look to God to know what he intended us to be. The late theologian Paul Jewett explains:

The truth that we have our being as human only in a fellowship of an I and a thou in no way impugns the distinction between them. True, I cannot rightly understand myself apart from God who gave me my existence and my neighbor with whom I share that existence. But the boundary between the self and the other is an ineluctable one. Hence Christian theology rejects all pantheistic, mystical merging of the creature with the Creator and recognizes, at the human level, the uniqueness and worth of the personal self over against all other selves.[3]

It is not presumptuous to see ourselves as unique, valuable individuals with a delegated authority over creation. God has given us what every human being so desperately seeks. Each of us wants to be loved and recognized as significant. Isaiah 43:1-3 reveals the extent to which God meets that human need for us:

But now thus says the LORD, he who created you, O Jacob, he who formed you, O Israel: Do not fear, for I have redeemed you; I have called you by name, you are mine. When you pass through the waters, I will be with you; and through the rivers, they shall not overwhelm you; when you walk through fire you shall not be burned, and the flame shall not consume you. For I am the LORD your God, the Holy One of Israel, your Savior.

In the face of sickness, death and other forms of distress, such an understanding of human existence provides the only satisfying explanation and offers the only real hope for the future. If we view ourselves merely as naturalistic beings who can control the physical environment at our will, we very quickly reach the limits of our powers. Science and technology bring us amazing capabilities, but they have yet to conquer death or rid the world of social problems. On the other hand, if we view ourselves as one with the universe, we are at the mercy of fate and the natural elements, with no basis for hope or for personal relationships.

We know that God is good, and since we reflect the image of God, humanity was created good—in fact, *very* good (Gen 1:31). But something happened to mar that image. It happened very soon after creation itself. For in creating us in his image, God also gave us the freedom to choose our own way over God's. By the third chapter of Genesis our first ancestors had already exercised that prerogative. We have been dealing with the consequences ever since, and repeating the same dysfunctional patterns generation after generation.

Hence, we cannot fully understand ourselves by empirical means alone. Nor can we know our true nature intuitively. Our observations and experience will always be colored by our fallen human nature. Not even science can be "value-free." The only way we can know what God intended us to be is to look at Jesus Christ. Hebrews 1:3 tells us that "he [Jesus] is the reflection of God's glory and the exact imprint of God's very being." Theologian Jürgen Moltmann asserts, "Christian anthropology is an anthropology of the crucified Lord: it is in relation to this 'son of man' that man recognizes his truth and first becomes true man."[4]

So what can we learn about ourselves and the persons entrusted to our care by looking at Jesus? First, we should be impressed that Jesus was a relational being. His relationship to God the Father is clearly described in Scripture, but he was also born into a very human family and community, and he saw himself as a citizen of both the kingdom of God and the political kingdom in which he resided. Second, Jesus demonstrated our multidimensional nature. By taking on human flesh, God reaffirmed the goodness of our physical bodies and human emotions without downplaying the importance of the spiritual aspect of our nature.

Third, Jesus showed us that we are sexual beings. He came as a man, "who in every respect has been tempted as we are, yet without sinning" (Heb 4:15 RSV). Yet he also raised the status of women and was not afraid to use female metaphors for God's actions toward his people (see, for example, Mt 23:37). Furthermore, Jesus demonstrated that God made us moral creatures who are to share God's love with our fellow creatures through ethical conduct and compassionate actions. Finally, Jesus showed us that we are mortals destined for eternal life. Even Jesus died, but he rose again in a new body that could not be destroyed.

Each of these characteristics of human existence holds profound implications for nursing. From them we draw our motivation for being nurses in the first place, but, more than that, they shape the nature of nursing itself. Em Olivia Bevis recognizes this fact by asserting, "Nursing works with people . . . and as such it is concerned with human welfare. To be concerned with human welfare is to act out of a belief in the worth of the individual and the worth of life."[5]

What we believe about human beings will determine how we treat one another. The Christian understanding of the person is that we are physically, psychosocially and spiritually integrated sexual, moral and mortal beings, created in God's image to live in relationship with God and others and as responsible stewards of the environment. If nurses lose sight of this understanding of human worth and human life, our profession will cease to exist, for there will no longer be any reason to provide nursing care. With this in mind we will investigate each of these aspects of human nature more carefully from a biblical perspective.

Relational Beings

Joe Blevins, age eighty and in relatively good health except for minor short-term memory loss, was admitted to the hospital for a stapedectomy. He expected to go home the next day, so he had his bags packed early that morning. When his son Bob arrived to get him, he explained to his father that the family could no longer care for him. So Joe would be going to a supervised group home instead of his familiar room at Bob's house. Joe reeled and stumbled into a nearby wheelchair, holding his head in his hands. "I don't feel good—get the nurse!" By the time the nurse arrived, only a few minutes later, Joe had spiked a fever of 104.6°F and seemed disoriented. He died of pneumonia three days later.

Mary Evans cared for her husband, Ken, as he grew increasingly debilitated from amyotrophic lateral sclerosis. Although exhausted from long hours of hard work, she maintained excellent health. After Ken's death, though, she began to catch every virus that went around. One Sunday morning during a blood pressure check, Mary told Susan, her parish nurse, that she didn't have any reason to live now that Ken was gone. Susan told Mary that she could use her help teaching a class for young people about living with disabilities. Mary didn't think she had the energy, but she agreed to try. Three weeks into the course she was a different person. The teenage class members appreciated Mary's listening ear and soon began to drop by her house just to talk. Some deep friendships began to develop. Mary eventually became involved with a local support group for people with ALS and their families.

God created human beings to live in community. When people lose that sense of love and belonging, they lose their meaning and purpose in life. Without this sense of hope, they lose their will to live, and they may even die without apparent cause. Most experienced nurses could tell too many stories like the ones above. On the other hand, most could tell stories about terminally ill patients who seemed to hang on against all odds until a son could return from overseas or a strained relationship could be repaired.

The most basic unit of relationships is the family. The family was God's idea, and it holds a high place throughout the Bible. Psalm 68:5-6 (NIV) tells us: "A father to the fatherless, a defender of widows, is God in his holy dwelling. God sets the lonely in families." A cursory look at the book of Genesis reveals that these families were far from perfect. The family is marred by the same sin that pervades every human heart. Adam and Eve established the world's first dysfunctional family, where sibling rivalry eventually escalated to murder. The generations that followed continued in patterns of conflict, deceit, manipulation and abuse. The Bible is strangely silent about how to deal with these dysfunctions. In fact, it almost seems as if God chose people we might label as narcissistic or borderline personalities for special honor and responsibility![6]

The biblical understanding of family went far beyond the nuclear family of today. Moses was an adopted child (Ex 2). Ruth, who became an ancestor of Jesus, was taken in by a distant relative of her late husband (Ruth 4). The Old Testament makes it very clear that the people of God were to care for those people who did not have families. For example, God expresses his concern for those who have no families in Deuteronomy 10:17-18, saying, "For the LORD your God is God of gods and Lord of lords . . . who executes justice for the orphan and the widow, and who loves the strangers, providing them food and clothing." In Deuteronomy 27:19 he instructs, "Cursed be anyone who deprives the alien, the orphan, and the widow of justice." This theme is repeated throughout the Old Testament.[7]

The New Testament expands the understanding of family to include the whole believing community. Jesus told his disciples, "For whoever does the will of my Father in heaven is my brother and sister and mother" (Mt 12:50) This theme of love and relatedness within the Christian community resonates throughout the New Testament. Jesus said:

I give you a new commandment, that you love one another. Just as I have loved you, you also should love one another. By this everyone will know that you are my disciples, if you have love for one another. (Jn 13:34-35)

However, throughout the New Testament we also see a clear recognition that this love will not come easily. The Gospels record how Jesus dealt with jealousy, prejudice, doubt, greed, abandonment, power ploys and abuse from both his friends and his enemies. He suffered greatly in the process: in the end he was executed by those who felt threatened by his love. The rest of the New Testament gives detailed instructions to Christians about how we are to live in loving relationship with one another, including how to deal with strained and broken relationships.

This love expanded beyond the Christian community to also include the neighbor. When asked by a skeptical lawyer, "Who is my neighbor?" Jesus replied with the story of the Good Samaritan (Lk 10:25-37). The neighbor in this case turned out to be a man of a different race, religion and social status who willingly provided compassionate care for an injured man.

What this means for us as nurses is that we cannot adequately care for people if we see them only as isolated individuals. We view each one in the context of families, communities and cultures. From this vantage point we can observe patterns that may contribute to illness or provide strength for healing. As we will see in chapter ten, human relationships are basic to a Christian understanding of health.

Multidimensional Beings

Brothers Fred and Wayne hardly spoke to one another. Both were active members of the same church. Both spoke easily of their deep faith to friends at work and in the neighborhood. But mention one brother's name to the other and you could see his face flush and his neck veins stand out. Always competitive with one another, their rivalry had grown ugly when Fred accused Wayne of taking more than his share of their parents' inheritance. Their pastor tried to encourage them to forgive each other, but each replied, "Never!" Within ten years both developed serious coronary artery disease and hypertension. They died of myocardial infarctions within a year of each other.

The psalmist described a similar interrelationship between spiritual and physical problems:

> While I kept silence, my body wasted away through my groaning all day long. For day and night your hand was heavy upon me; my strength was dried up as by the heat of summer. Then I acknowledged my sin to you, and I did not hide my iniquity; I said, "I will confess my transgressions to the LORD," and you forgave the guilt of my sin. (Ps 32:3-5)

Central to both the Old and New Testaments is the understanding of the person as an integrated whole. There is no body-mind dualism. Instead there is a vibrant sense of the person in relationship to God and the world through the bodily senses and functions.

First let's look at the Old Testament. In order to understand Hebrew terms, we must get inside the Semitic mind, keeping in mind two significant points. First, concepts like "heart," "soul," "flesh" and "spirit" are often interchangeable in Hebrew thought. Second, Hebrew thinking is stereometric, simultaneously presupposing "a synopsis of the members and organs of the human body with their capacities and functions."[8] In other words, often when a part of the body is mentioned, its function is implied.[9]

The Hebrew term *nēpeš* refers to the person in need and encompasses everything from throat and neck to desire, soul, life and the person as a whole. *Bāśār*, while referring to the body or flesh, essentially means the person in relationship and the person in weakness. *Rûaḥ*, referring to wind, breath, vital powers, spirit, feeling and will, describes the person as empowered. Hence the individual does not *have* a body, soul or spirit, but *is* all of those things at once. *Lēḇ* is the reasonable, thinking person, and it is tied to the heart. Ultimately the individual is always viewed in relationship.

The Hebrew concept of the human being provides a solid foundation for nursing theory and practice. Nursing is concerned about the whole person and how persons interrelate to maintain and restore health. For the Hebrew, health was found in a dynamic relationship with Yahweh. Sickness was both a physical and a spiritual problem that warranted not only hygienic practices but also self-examination, confession and prayer.

The New Testament also views the person in relationship to God as a total being. For instance, Paul closes his first letter to the Thessalonians by praying, "May the God of peace himself sanctify you entirely; and may your spirit and soul and body be kept sound and blameless at the coming of our Lord Jesus Christ" (1 Thess 5:23). Here he is speaking in the common Hebrew form of parallelism, repeating the same thought in different words. Rather than suggesting that people have three distinct parts (spirit, soul, body), he is simply referring to the sanctification of the whole person.

The most comprehensive New Testament term characterizing the person's total existence is the Greek word *sōma* (body).[10] A person does not have a *sōma*, but is *sōma*, just as in the Old Testament a person does not have a *nēpeš*, but is *nēpeš*. In a similar way, the terms *psychē* (soul, or life itself) and *pneuma* (spirit) are used by Paul to designate the person as a whole. When the terms are used in conjunction with one another, such as in 1 Thessalonians 5:23, they are intended to summarize the totality of a human being.[11] Furthermore, the terms heart (*kardia*) and mind (*nous*) are largely synonymous and designate the person as a "willing, planning, intending self."[12]

The body, soul, mind, spirit and even the various body parts are expressions of the wholeness that is the human self. They designate the whole person as seen from different perspectives. All of these aspects are summed up in the term *zōē:* life that is given by God and makes the person the subject of his or her own actions.[34]

While this view does not divide the person into unrelated parts, it does allow for distinctions. A corpse is not a person because the *psychē* (in this case *life*) has departed from it. Our bodies are the way we experience life and relate to the world. But we are embodied spirits (or souls), and, to some degree, the spiritual takes preeminence over the physical. After death we will not be left disembodied, but be raised in "spiritual bodies" (1 Cor 15:35-57). Jewett explains:

> When used of the human creature, "spirit" refers to that vital principle which animates the body and enables one to feel, think, will, and desire. As such, it is the seat of psychic experience and has essentially the same meaning as "soul" *(yuch)*. Being the seat of psychic experience, the human spirit is especially engaged as one relates to God.[14]

This view of the person is quite different from that of New Paradigm theorists who describe the person as an energy field with no distinctions between body and spirit. In that understanding, the body is merely an illusion or a lump of "congealed energy."

The New Paradigm energy theory comes with two problematic implications. First, it assumes that the energy of each person is the same energy that makes up the universe. Hence, New Paradigm nurses may claim that we are really gods and goddesses—but at the same time, we are one with the frogs and rocks and trees. There are no distinctions between persons and the rest of the universe any more than there are distinctions within a person. Second, it assumes that the spiritual is the only reality; hence, advocates desire to escape the physical body through spiritual cultivation—meditation and certain spiritual disciplines. On a lesser scale, the mind (soul/spirit) becomes the means of healing the physical body through manipulating energy fields.

The Bible teaches that God is not just an energy field, and neither are we. Although God creates people in his image, we remain creatures; we are not divine, we are not part of God. The body is the temple of the Holy Spirit.[15] God enters his people to enliven and inspire them, but we are not God and cannot become gods. However, God is both transcendent and immanent. In Isaiah 57:15 God says,

> For thus says the high and lofty one
>   who inhabits eternity, whose name is Holy:
> I dwell in the high and holy place,
>   and also with those who are contrite and
>   humble in spirit,
> to revive the spirit of the humble,
>   and to revive the heart of the contrite.

God relates to us as a Father to his children (Mt 6:8; 7:11; Lk 12:32). In fact, through Jesus Christ, God became human in order to "sympathize with our weaknesses" (Heb 4:15).

Sexual Beings

Perhaps it is in our sexuality that we experience our human weakness most acutely. Most of us know sexual temptation; we must deal with sexual discrimination; all too often we see the broken lives that result from sexual abuse. But sex is good. Not only did God create us as sexual beings, but Scripture actually uses the sexual relationship as an analogy for God's relationship to us.

Mystics in years gone by reveled in the sexual images of God, seeing God as a divine Lover. We are a bit more prudish today. Our understanding of sex has been warped by sin, just as our relationship with God is marred.

Studying sexuality can teach us more about God's love for us.

Paul uses an analogy in Ephesians 5:

> For no one ever hates his own body, but he nourishes and tenderly cares for it, just as Christ does for the church, because we are members of his body. "For this reason a man will leave his father and mother and be joined to his wife, and the two will become one flesh." This is a great mystery, and I am applying it to Christ and the church. (vv. 29-32)

Here we see that, just as the marriage relationship brings a man and a woman together in a total way, so Jesus draws us to himself and cares for us completely. We are not his individual lovers, but part of a body (the church) that is called "the bride of Christ." We must be a functioning part of that body in order to relate to God fully. But then, we see that our relationship with God naturally should be charged with passion and emotion. It should be characterized by a deep desire to please him and to enjoy him. There is a sense of permanence and exclusivity. Nothing should be able to woo us away from our loving God.

God is deeply hurt by our unfaithfulness. He vividly demonstrated his pain in the book of Hosea when he told the prophet to marry a prostitute named Gomer. Gomer did not change her ways, and Hosea constantly grieved over her unfaithfulness and its disastrous effects on their family. When he had Hosea's full attention, God explained how the pain and destructiveness of Gomer's behavior related to Israel's and Judah's idolatry.

The analogy works the other way around, too. We can learn about good sex from examining God's relationship with us. It is based on unselfish love. He is willing to sacrifice anything for us, even his own Son. His commitment does not waver, despite our weak faith and roaming eyes.

Genesis 1:27 tells us: "God created humankind in his image, in the image of God he created them; male and female he created them." It is no accident that we are both male and female. They are two complementary aspects of God's nature. His image is not complete in one gender alone. We need each other. That does not mean that everyone has to be married to be complete. Instead, we need to think and work together. Both all-male and all-female living or working situations tend to lead toward distortions of the way God intended us to live.

Later in Genesis we read, "Now the man knew his wife Eve, and she conceived" (4:1). The verb *to know* is not just a Hebrew euphemism for sexual intercourse. In Hosea 13:5 (RSV) God says, "It was I who knew you in the wilderness." Then he describes his commitment to love, nourish and heal. "It is I who answer and look after you. I am like an evergreen cypress, from me comes your fruit" (14:8 RSV). Genital sexuality is always placed in the context of absolute commitment. And the fruit of that union brings further commitment to care for it properly.

Sexuality is a mystery designed to bring pleasure, joy, security and purpose into the relationship between husband and wife. It is a small glimpse of life in heaven where the church is the bride of Christ. But for all that is good about sex, we live in a fallen world. Even stable marriages can be rocky at times. We are bombarded with messages that sex is an expected part of casual relationships. The old-fashioned idea of keeping sex within marriage is widely regarded as impractical, even by many committed Christians. The threat of disease—AIDS, genital herpes, venereal warts, resistant strains of syphilis and gonorrhea—has spread fear but not significantly changed behavior. Why should anyone be different? Why be chaste?

First, because sex outside of marriage violates our God-given desire for a faithful sexual relationship. It destroys trust and deflates hope and self-esteem. Even between engaged couples, sex can become overpowering and manipulative. It can prevent them from getting to know one another well enough to build a solid marriage.[16]

Second, casual sex reduces intercourse to genital pleasure instead of letting it be the sign of absolute love and commitment it was intended to be. When that basic need is not met, sex can become an addiction, a desperate search for the ultimate high. The average adult in the United States has had seven sexual partners. Many gay men have had *thousands* of encounters.[17] Addictions become idols. They pull us away from God and become the center around which our lives are organized.

Finally, sexual sin is passed on to the generations that follow us. We are experiencing the crisis of a generation of children who come from dysfunctional homes. Many have had to adjust to a constant flow of changing stepparents or parents' live-in lovers. They have never seen faithfulness demonstrated in their families. With no model of a loving human father, is it any wonder that they show no interest in God the Father?

Because God created us as sexual beings, good nursing must include working toward sexual health. Sexual function cannot be divided into a separate compartment, any more than nutrition, hydration or exercise can. Sexual behavior affects not only a person's physical health but also self-image, interpersonal relationships and relationship with God. Poor choices of sexual partners and practices may affect a person's entire future. The high-school honor student who becomes pregnant may have to give up plans for college. Another who ends her pregnancy in abortion may suffer a lifetime of guilt and shame. Sexually transmitted diseases may result in a lifetime of anguish or even death.

What does good nursing include for people who because of disability, illness, sexual orientation or marital status cannot experience genital sex? First of all, we need to acknowledge that this is a painful loss. Second, we can help such people to find their ultimate meaning and significance in God rather than in the sexual experience. However, all people still need human intimacy. We can offer and encourage appropriate caring touch and also give practical counsel on how to deal with sexual feelings.

Sexuality encompasses the physical, emotional and spiritual aspects of our being. Therefore, simplistic campaigns such as "safe sex" (advocating condoms to prevent venereal disease) or encouraging birth control to prevent pregnancy in single women do not truly promote sexual health. Sexual health involves engaging a person's total being in expressing sexuality—with or without sexual activity—according to God's plan in creation. It also includes an understanding of the role of gender in human relationships and an appreciation of the differences between men and women.

Moral Beings

As sexuality only too clearly reminds us, God also created us to be moral beings. The fact that there are some boundaries around our sexual behavior implies that we must make moral choices. While the boundaries seem to be shifting much faster in today's world and the expanding choices may feel overwhelming, the problem is not new. The human struggle with morality began in the Garden of Eden.

> The LORD God took the man and put him in the garden of Eden to till it and keep it. And the LORD God commanded the man, "You may freely eat of every tree of the garden; but of the tree of the knowledge of good and evil you shall not eat, for in the day that you eat of it you shall die." (Gen 2:15-17)
>
> Now the serpent was more crafty than any other wild animal that the LORD God had made. He said to the woman, "Did God say, 'You shall not eat from any tree in the garden'?" The woman said to the serpent, "We may eat of the fruit of the trees in the garden; but God said, 'You shall not eat of the fruit of the tree that is in the middle of the garden, nor shall you touch it, or you shall die.'" But the serpent said to the woman, "You will not die; for God knows that when you eat of it your eyes will be opened, and you will be like God, knowing good and evil." So when the woman saw that the tree was good for food, and that it was a delight to the eyes, and that the tree was to be desired to make one wise, she took of its fruit and ate; and she also gave some to her husband, who was with her, and he ate. (Gen 3:1-6)

Played out right here in the very beginning, we can see the same tensions that we face today. God set a moral boundary. The serpent challenged it and convinced the woman to cross it. In the process, she moved from ethical absolutism to ethical relativism. But even then she did not reject morality entirely. She used an ethical decision-making process based on what was *good*. She rationalized that the good she saw through her own reasoning outweighed the good that God intended, and then she acted on her decision.

That moral sense is what separates human beings from the rest of the animals. Although the perception of what is good or just may differ from culture to culture and even from person to person, we are all born with some sense of fairness and a need for rules. Those who refuse to live by those moral boundaries are considered immoral.

Dogs, frogs and amoebas cannot be immoral. If I leave my sandwich within range of my cocker spaniel and turn my back, she will grab it and disappear. I may yell "Bad dog!" at her, and she will sulk in a corner because she has displeased me, but she is not immoral. However, if I leave my wallet on the table, and my friend steals a $20 bill while I am not looking, she has committed an immoral act. We even use different language for human behavior. We don't accuse horses of lying, cheating, stealing, jealousy, murder, idolatry or unfaithfulness. That is the language of human moral codes, including the Ten Commandments (Ex 20:1-17).

The problem of good and evil has occupied philosophers from the beginning of time. What makes the question so consuming is that the problem is not just in the external world—it is within us. The apostle Paul describes the dilemma this way:

> So I find it to be a law that when I want to do what is good, evil lies close at hand. For I delight in the law of God in my inmost self, but I see in my members another law at war with the law of my mind, making me captive to the law of sin that dwells in my members. Wretched man that I am! Who will rescue me from this body of death? (Rom 7:21-24)

The question of morality looms large for nurses, because our profession claims to be doing good for others. Nursing puts us face to face with issues and situations that demand a moral response. We have to know what the good is before we can do it, and the answers are not clearly evident.

For example, during a rather intense ethical discussion, a frustrated nursing student shouted, "Don't give me alternatives; just tell me the Christian position!" She was not the first one to feel that way. Ethical decision-making always puts us in an awkward situation. We are usually forced to choose the least-worst alternative, for there are seldom purely good solutions.

It would be nice if there were a clear Christian position on all the questions we face about life, death and morality. We wouldn't have to wrestle with gut-wrenching decisions or study ethics. We could just check out the manual on Christian positions, find the answer and go about our business. Some Christians have tried to make the Bible into such a manual, but it doesn't really provide us with clear directions about when to remove a ventilator, or the morality of mapping human genomes, or even an absolute definition of death.

The Bible does give us some absolutes by which to make ethical decisions. The Ten Commandments lay down the basics: faithfulness to God, keeping the Sabbath, honoring our parents, protecting life, sexual purity, respecting private property, honesty, and being content with what we have. Jesus summarized the commandments by saying, "'You shall love the Lord your God with all your heart, and with all your soul, and with all your mind.' This is the greatest and first commandment. And a second is like it: 'You shall love your neighbor as yourself.' On these two commandments hang all the law and the prophets" (Mt 22:37-40).

Being a moral Christian in the real world isn't easy. The line between life and death is often blurred. New technology makes old definitions of death obsolete. The twentieth century has compounded the problem with the frantic pace of technological development, but the problem is not new. Hymn writer James Russell Lowell (1819-1891) put it well:

New occasions teach new duties;
time makes ancient good uncouth;
they must upward still and onward,
who would keep abreast of truth.

Truth doesn't change, but the context does. Our moral nature makes us strive to do good.

In a society lost in a sea of relativism, people are desperate for absolutes. Even those without a strong Christian faith are beginning to be alarmed by the "if it feels good, do it" philosophy that has guided American ethics for the past several decades. When voters must decide whether physicians should be permitted to kill their patients, something is drastically wrong!

Many Christians are grasping for a solid dividing line between the morally acceptable and the unacceptable, fearing the slippery slope into antinomianism (lawlessness).[18] In the process, we have sometimes alienated or excommunicated one another, refusing to respect one another's decisions or methods of decision-making. At such times we can take hope in the understanding that God has created us as moral beings who, though corrupted by sin, still have an innate sense of justice and goodness.

Mortal Beings

We are both *moral* and *mortal*. We struggle with questions of life and death. The preacher in Ecclesiastes tells us, "For everything there is a season, and a time for every matter under heaven: a time to be born, and a time to die" (3:1-2).

We don't like to face our mortality. People have been seeking the "Fountain of Youth" from the beginning of time. Most of us deny our own mortality. Recently, a friend close to my age and I (Judy) struggled to stand up after sitting on the floor to watch a video. As I reached to assist her, she remarked, "I guess we're just feeling the effects of middle age." Suddenly the irony of her statement struck me. Although the definition of "middle age" seems to be getting progressively older as I age, I seriously doubt that I will live to be over 100!

Middle-class American culture clings to the hope in "progress" when it comes to death. If diet, exercise and cosmetics can't hold death at bay, certainly medical technology will save us. We hide people who are dying in medical centers or nursing homes, and we bury those who have "passed on," their appearances improved by make-up, in what are sometimes called "memorial gardens." We thereby lose sight of our personal mortality—the fact that we will one day *die*. In this we tend to be an anomaly in human history and culture.

In former times, and in many cultures today, people died at home, surrounded by family and friends. As a teenager I (Judy) remember my Great-Uncle Otto lying in state in the parlor of his home. We sat around eating meals, telling family stories, even laughing. My father's sister shuddered as she confided, "Every time I walk into this room I think of death." I had to agree that it felt a bit strange to be enjoying ourselves with Uncle Otto's body laid out in the open casket, but is it so bad that we were forced to think about death?

My own church building was constructed because the farmers in this rural area wanted a place to bury their dead. Today we complain that there is no room to expand because we cannot move the graves. But there is also a sense of continuity with the saints who have died in the Lord. Some of the older members have already erected their tombstones in anticipation of their own deaths. That is a healthy sense of human mortality.

We are mortals, but God has given us eternal life in Jesus Christ. We die, and yet we live. That is but one of the tensions that we embrace as Christians. We will explore the concept of death more fully in chapter twelve, but here let us briefly summarize the implications of this mortality for nursing.

First, all human beings will die. Many of our patients will die in our care, but those deaths do not necessarily mean we have failed. Freed from the anxiety to preserve physical life at all costs, we can offer comfort, care and hope in the face of death.

On the other hand, poor stewardship of the life God has given us may well exacerbate the death and decay that surround us. Poor diets, lack of exercise, substance abuse, environmental pollutants, dysfunctional relationships and a host of other irresponsible human actions, including assisted suicide, may hasten death. But God has instructed us:

> I have set before you life and death, blessings and curses. Choose life so that you and your descendants may live, loving the LORD your God, obeying him, and holding fast to him; for that means life to you and length of days. (Deut 30:19-20)

As nurses who are mortal human beings, we have committed ourselves to choosing life in its fullness for ourselves and those in our care. We work toward health and healing. We fight death as an enemy. At the same time we recognize our limitations, knowing that we are not able to control all circumstances, but remaining confident that we can know and trust the One who does.

Being human makes us glorious beings who reflect the nature of God. We are thinking, feeling, willful beings, embodied spirits who are moral and mortal. Although God created us to live in relationship with himself, we struggle with sin and are constantly rebelling against God and wounding our neighbors. Yet God restores us to himself through Jesus Christ. In Jesus we find our true humanity, freeing us to love and care for others.

5

The Person as a Spiritual Being

ANNA MOANED IN PAIN. SHE WAS THREE DAYS POST-OP FROM removal of abdominal adhesions, and everything indicated that she was healing well, but the pain continued. Nothing seemed to help. I (Judy) had given her all the PRN analgesics she could have and called her physician to have the dosage increased. He refused. I tried rubbing her back, bringing her a cup of tea and turning her radio to some soothing music. Still her muscles tightened in agony. "Why does God allow me to suffer so?" She moaned, "He must hate me!"

From her clenched fist dangled a crucifix on a rosary. A brainstorm struck me. "Do you think God hated *him*?" I asked, pointing to the crucifix.

"Of course not—he *was* God!" Anna replied.

We continued to talk about God's love for us being demonstrated in the cross of Christ. Then I offered to pray for her. Afterward, Anna's muscles slowly relaxed and the pain eased. She slept through the night.

While most nurses would quickly acknowledge that Anna's pain stemmed from more than physical causes at this point, they would probably attribute it to psychological factors. However, Anna's problem was spiritual. Further discussions with her revealed a complicated web of broken family relationships and a painful estrangement from her church. Anna harbored a deep anger toward her former husband, her son, the church and God. She figured that God must hate her as well.

My friend Martha would have a different approach, although her assessment of the problem would be similar. I met Martha at a nursing convention and liked her immediately. A devout Roman Catholic, Martha taught a course on therapeutic touch and other alternative therapies in her church-related college nursing program. She enthusiastically described how these energy-based therapies brought marked relief almost every time she used them.

After listening for several minutes, I finally asked her about the source of the energy she believed she was channeling. "Oh, it's the Holy Spirit!" she said happily.

As I probed further, it became apparent that she was working from an eclectic worldview. In typical Western fashion she had put her Christian beliefs into the category of "religion" but somehow reserved a pragmatic area for what she called "spirituality," which could be related to her nursing practice. For Martha spirituality dwelt in the worldview of monistic energy fields which she envisioned as the Holy Spirit.

"It makes me kind of nervous to think of trying to manipulate God," I replied, trying to gently move her toward thinking about the implications of what she was doing.

"But we are *supposed* to be channels of the Holy Spirit," she continued, "It's just the laying on of hands with another name."

It soon became apparent that our conversation might quickly degenerate into a fruitless argument, so we changed the subject. However, Martha kept coming back to talk more. By the end of the week we were friends. Although we respected each other, neither of us changed the other's mind.

What differentiates the spiritual from the physical or psychological? We have already established that these aspects are not separate parts of a person, but that they can be distinguished. Our dualistic Western culture would like to see the spiritual as either nonexistent or irrelevant. It would say that Anna's pain should be controlled with the proper medical or surgical intervention, or at least a psychiatric consultation if all else failed. In this worldview reality is essentially physical or material. However, in the face of

Anna's very real pain, the spiritual dimension had to be addressed in order to bring relief.

On the other hand, Martha and other proponents of new spiritualities would argue that the heart of *all* Anna's problems was spiritual, and that they could be corrected by techniques to balance her universal energy flow. Although most advocates of the new spiritualities also use Western allopathic remedies, they do so with reluctance. In this worldview reality is essentially spiritual.

In the Christian worldview, spirituality is essentially relationship—a relationship of the whole person to a personal God and to other people (or other spirits). The spiritual is always personal. It is not an impersonal energy force. The personal nature of spirituality imbues it with deep moral and ethical implications. Dallas Willard explains, "Spirituality is simply the holistic quality of human life as it was meant to be, at the center of which is our relation to God."[1] He further elaborates, "the spiritual is a homogeneous aspect, part and parcel of the biological (and therefore social) nature of human beings."[2]

Spirituality in Nursing

The nursing literature reflects our culture's changing understanding of spirituality. Although earlier definitions attempted to differentiate spirituality from religion, most saw spirituality as involving a person's relationship with God, while later references began to view it as a life principle.

Joan Haase et al. attempted to synthesize the definitions of spirituality in the nursing literature. They came to the conclusion that while *spirituality* was consistently seen as a basic or inherent quality of all human beings, what differed was *spiritual perspective*, which they defined as "a highly individualized awareness of one's spirituality and its qualities." They found three critical attributes of spiritual perspective: (1) connectedness (with others, nature, the universe or God), (2) belief (in something greater than the self), and (3) creative energy "that is in constant, yet dynamic, evolutionary flux."[3]

Based on these attributes, they defined spiritual perspective as "an integrating and creative energy based on a belief in, and a feeling of interconnectedness with, a power greater than self." Their literature review also found three apparent outcomes of spirituality: (1) purpose and meaning, (2) guidance of human values and (3) self-transcendence.[4] However, the worldviews inherent in the articles they surveyed were not differentiated, so that they merely combined and summarized incompatible spiritual perspectives.

Using concept analysis Emblen investigated the terms *spiritual* and *spirituality* in the nursing literature, comparing them with the concept of *religion*. In definitions of *religion* six terms appeared most frequently: *system, beliefs, organized, person, worship* and *practices*. On the other hand, *spirituality* was associated with the terms *personal, life, principle, animator, being, God (god), quality, relationship* and *transcendent*. By using these terms to form consensus definitions, Emblen concluded that *spirituality* is a broader term that may include some aspects of religion. However, she also notes that "the term *spiritual* is rapidly acquiring new and varied definitions."[5]

An earlier study by Burkhardt summarized definitions of terms related to spirituality, showing a wide variation but concluding that "spirituality goes beyond a focus on religiosity" and "spiritual care needs to be based on a more universal concept of inspiriting rather than religion or religiosity."[6] She further concludes, quoting from Viktor Frankl:

> The concept of spiriting has no antecedents. Spiriting is "a thing in itself. It cannot be explained by something not spiritual; it is irreducible. It may be conditioned by something without being caused by it."[7]

If such is the case, the idea of a generic, broadly defined spirituality raises serious concerns for the Christian nurse. The spiritual world is not neutral, as most nursing authors seem to imply. The Bible makes it quite clear that when we seek a spirituality apart from the Spirit of God, we invite evil spirits to dwell in us (Mt 12:43-45; Col 2:8; Eph 5:6-17; 1 Tim 4:1).

Willard explains that there are two directions that spirituality can take in today's culture, Christian or "general human interest." He further clarifies:

> Much of modern thinking views spirituality as simply a kind of "interiority"—the idea that there is an inside to the human being, and

that is the place where contact is made with the transcendental. In this view, spirituality is essentially a human dimension.

Christian spirituality is centered in the idea of a transcendent life—"being born from above," as the New Testament puts it. This idea of the spiritual life carries with it the notions like accountability, judgment, the need for justice, and so on. These concepts are less popular, and they are certainly more difficult, than a conception of spirituality that simply focuses on one's inner life.[8]

In other words, secular spirituality is an aspect of human nature to be nurtured. It may include human relationships, but it is usually an inner experience. According to Steve Turner, "As used in secular discourse, *spiritual* can refer to anything that cannot either be tested in a laboratory or bolted to the floor."[9] On the other hand, the Bible presents spirituality as an encounter with a spiritual being separate from ourselves—either God or an evil spirit. Christian spirituality is essentially a personal relationship with God. Turner explains,

> Christian conversion is not a case of fanning that little spiritual spark in the human soul into a flame. It is a case of invading a dark and doomed soul with spiritual light from above.
>
> Christian spirituality does not originate in a small area of the human brain. It is a transference of God's personality into the human life, and it can only happen on the basis of repentance, faith, and discipleship. It cannot be coaxed, kick-started, or chanted into being. The original temptation is that we can become divine through a mechanical act.[10]

Martin Luther reacted strongly against the mystics of his day, believing that "enthusiasm" (in its technical sense of being inspired or possessed by a god) was the essence of original sin.[11] Salvation must come from without.

The Christian Spiritual Tradition

The Christian church does have a rich mystical tradition, which became suppressed during the Enlightenment and the rise of empiricism. We affirm that there is much in this tradition that should be restored and enjoyed.

Mysticism unchecked, however, frequently leads to serious heresy and corruption in the church and blurs the uniqueness of the Christian gospel. Psychologist Elizabeth Hillstrom points out that mystical writers from Maharishi Mahesh Yogi to Christian mystics like St. John of the Cross all warn about the dangers of "madness, demonic deception or possession for those who venture into the mystical path."[12] Richard Foster describes the goal of true Christian mysticism:

> In meditative prayer there is no loss of identity, no merging with the cosmic consciousness, no fanciful astral travel. Rather, we are called to life-transforming obedience because we have encountered the living God of Abraham, Isaac, and Jacob. Christ is truly present among us to heal us, to forgive us, to change us, to empower us.[13]

The Bible is the central reference point in Christian mysticism. The mystical experience must always be tested by the Scriptures, not the other way around. When mysticism moves beyond biblical limits, it ceases to be Christian, even when Christian terminology is retained.

In reviewing the history of Christian spirituality, George Lane defines spirituality as "man's possession by God in Christ through the Holy Spirit."[14] We first see this understanding of spirituality demonstrated by Jesus as he prays in John 17:

> And for their sakes I sanctify myself, so that they also may be sanctified in truth. I ask not only on behalf of these, but also on behalf of those who will believe in me through their word, that they may all be one. As you, Father, are in me and I am in you, may they also be in us, so that the world may believe that you have sent me. (vv. 19-21)

In this context Jesus is not referring to "oneness" as a monistic merging with God but as a dynamic personal relationship that results in a oneness of purpose and a reflection of Christ's character in his followers. This understanding of "union" or "oneness" with God is what separates Christian spirituality from all others.

Monism, the belief that "all is one," has challenged Christian faith from the very beginning. The early church faced attacks and subtle corruption by

Gnosticism (teaching that salvation was obtained through a secret knowledge) and Platonic philosophy (which sought salvation through ascetic practices and mystical experiences). Both of those influences taught a spiritual monism—that each person had a "divine spark," or a pure soul, that was imprisoned by a corrupt body. The goal of each divine spark was to shed the confines of the evil body to be rejoined with God. Both the Gnosticism of New Testament times and the later Neo-Platonism (third through sixth centuries) incorporated magic and sorcery. The early church fathers were unanimous in pointing to Simon the Magician in Acts 8 as the first Gnostic.[15] We see further evidence of these influences in many of the concerns that New Testament writers express to first-century churches in the Epistles.

Monism is an assumption that there is one eternal principle in the cosmos. It therefore denies a Creator above and separate from creation. It began around the sixth century B.C. in India and China, gradually spreading to Persia and later to Europe.[16] It appeared in various forms, such as Hinduism, Taoism, Buddhism, Gnosticism and Neo-Platonism. Today we see it reappearing in New Age religions. The appeal of monism comes from its assumption that all is One, and therefore all is God. This makes everyone God, removing all external ethical constraints. It is also highly experiential, seeking mystical union with God through meditation, dreams and visions. This experience then becomes the source of truth for the monist.

Historically, when Christians practiced mysticism, monism often followed; church leaders from Paul to Luther made strong efforts to control it. Mysticism refers to "the immediate experience of a divine-human relationship, and in particular to the experiences of oneness with a divine . . . being or state."[17] Prophecy, in the sense of delivering an inspired message from God, is a form of mysticism. We see this in Acts 21 when Paul visited Philip, an evangelist in Caesarea who was one of the seven appointed in Acts 6 to care for the Hellenistic Christians. Apparently his home was a center of mystical spirituality. Philip had four unmarried daughters who prophesied. During Paul's visit another prophet, Agabus, came and prophesied with great emotion that Paul would be imprisoned if he traveled on to Jerusalem. Paul, who experienced mystical visions and charismatic gifts himself (see in particular 1 Cor 12—14), refused to heed the prophet's message, even though it proved correct in the end. The New Testament and early Christian writings, such as the *Didache* (second century) set firm limits on the authority of anyone claiming to have gained knowledge through mystical means (Mt 7:15; 24:24; 1 Cor 14:37-40; 2 Pet 2:1-3; 1 Jn 4:1-6).

Several significant periods in church history produced outbreaks of mysticism—what many would call *spirituality* today. The first evidence came in the book of Acts and continued through the second and early third centuries. It was a time of intense persecution, and God seems to have provided powerful experiences to give the young church the encouragement and sense of mission to survive and grow in a hostile environment. Outstanding mystics from this period included Origen (185-254), an influential teacher in the early church, and Montanus, founder of a prophetic movement that began about 170. Origen was a brilliant scholar who struggled to reconcile his Christian faith with Greek philosophy. He was strongly influenced by Neo-Platonism but tried to use it in the service of Christian doctrine. The flamboyant cult leader Montanus, along with his female disciples Prisca and Maximilla, claimed to speak for the Holy Spirit while in ecstatic states.[18] Both met with strong criticism from the church, yet both also contributed to the rich history of the church's mystical tradition.

In the fourth century a new type of spirituality developed. Christianity had become the state religion with the conversion of Constantine. The church was corrupt, politicized and spiritually weak. The "desert fathers," including Anthony the Hermit, sought union with God by fleeing to the Egyptian desert to be away from the distractions of the world. These monks lived alone in the desert, often exhibiting bizarre behavior (extreme fasting, refusing to bathe, living at the top of tall pillars), but they were often visited by Christians seeking divine guidance, healing or deliverance from evil spirits. Some of these monks moved away from orthodox Christian teachings and into monism as they became consumed with mystical experiences and the contemplative life.

As life in the desert grew increasingly difficult, many of the monks began to cluster in monasteries. By the sixth century these monastic orders, under the influence of Benedict, became less focused on personal sanctification and more concerned about community life and reaching out to the world in charity and evangelism. One shining light for nursing in the twelfth century, Hildegard of Bingen, came from the Benedictine community. A spiritual leader and visionary who was also an expert in the use of herbs and midwifery, she wrote two books on healing.[19] By the thirteenth century the mendicant orders, led by the Dominicans and Franciscans, lived a common life with the explicit purpose of going out into the world to serve and to preach the gospel. They attempted to balance spirituality and service.

Overshadowed by the horrors of the Black Death, the Hundred Years War and scandalous corruption in the church, the fourteenth and fifteenth centuries produced a new round of mystical spirituality. The most famous Rhineland mystic of this period, Meister Eckhart, taught a mystical union with God in the neoplatonic tradition and was condemned by the church for "pantheism."[20] A bright light in this period was Julian of Norwich, an English mystic with a vibrant relationship with God. Her deep faith led her to reach out in compassion to others. Although Julian, as an anchoress, was not allowed to leave her "anchorhold" (a few rooms by a church), she would counsel local people through her window from behind a curtain.[21]

The sixteenth century was a time of tremendous turmoil in the church. It produced activist reformers like Martin Luther, John Calvin, Ulrich Zwingli, John Knox, Thomas Müntser and Conrad Grebel. This period also produced some of the most influential mystics, such as Ignatius of Loyola, Teresa of Ávila and John of the Cross. The activists and the contemplatives did not understand each other. While Luther ranted against enthusiasm, Teresa of Ávila prayed for him, asking God to "give light to the Lutherans."[22]

This rift between the Reformers and the mystics resulted in a long suspicion of the contemplative tradition in most Protestant churches. Their reasons for concern were not without cause. Many of the mystics, such as the Spanish Illuminati, believed that once they had reached mystical union with God they no longer had to heed any other authority. Ignatius countered that the union one should seek with God was not a matter of cosmic merging that rendered a person ethically autonomous, but a correspondence to the divine will. His spiritual disciplines and the writings of Teresa of Ávila and John of the Cross provide great inspiration to Christians today who are seeking a deeper spirituality.

Spirituality in the Bible

Postmodern people today are reacting against the emptiness of modern religion. Too often liberal Christianity has taught that true religion is doing the right things.[23] Evangelicals have tended to focus on believing the right doctrines.[24] Neither has fed the deep hunger most people feel for intimacy with God, leaving seekers disillusioned and often angry. The postmodern alternative to organized religion is a contentless, experiential spirituality— what we are calling *generic spirituality*. Interestingly, the term *spirituality* does not appear anywhere in the Bible, nor does the abstract concept of spirituality. However, several Hebrew and Greek terms are translated as *spirit* or *spiritual* in the Bible. If we consider spirituality to be that which pertains to the spiritual realm, then a brief study of these words should inform our definition of Christian spirituality.

The first appearance of the word *spirit* in the Old Testament comes in Genesis 1. It is the Hebrew term *rûaḥ*, which the NRSV translates in this case as "a wind from God." The same term is used in Genesis 2:7: "then the LORD God formed man from the dust of the ground, and breathed into his nostrils the *breath of life*; and the man became a living being." According to Old Testament scholar Hans Walter Wolff, *rûaḥ* is used in six different ways in the Old Testament: wind, breath, vital powers, spirit(s), feelings and will.[25] When used in relation to humans, *rûaḥ* refers to the person as empowered by God. It is always under God's control, not something humans possess. However, it is the *rûaḥ* of God that communicates with the human *rûaḥ* in dynamic relationship. Wolff explains, "a man as *rûaḥ* is living, desires the good and acts as authorized being—none of this proceeds from man himself."[26]

The equivalent term for *rûaḥ* in the New Testament is the Greek word *pneuma*. It can mean wind, breath or "that dimension of the human personality whereby relationship with God is possible."[27] It may also refer to disembodied created beings, as well as to God himself. In two cases Paul refers to those who are *spiritual* as Christians who are mature in Christ (1 Cor 3:1; Gal 6:1), but nowhere do we see him urging his followers to develop their *spirituality*. Instead the New Testament focuses on seeking God through Christ and doing his will. Jesus taught his disciples the importance of prayer, and the spiritual gifts certainly play an important role throughout the New Testament; however, their purpose is centered in restoring humanity's broken relationship with God. They are evidence of God's in-breaking kingdom (Lk 4:18), preparing his people to move out into the world proclaiming good news to the poor, liberty to the captives, sight to the blind and freedom for the oppressed.

The Bible takes for granted that an unseen spiritual world exists. Throughout the Old Testament, God warned his people to avoid any dealings with spirits other than himself (Ex 20:1-6; Lev 19:31; Deut 18:9-14; 1 Sam 28:3-19; 1 Chron 10:13-14). The entire history of Israel provides graphic stories of the personal disintegration and national corruption that resulted when God's people violated this command. In the New Testament, Jesus began his ministry by going into the wilderness, where he was tempted by Satan and attended by angels (Mt 4:1-11; Mk 1:12-13; Lk 4:1-13). Throughout his ministry he confronted evil spirits; furthermore, he commissioned his followers to teach, preach and cast out demons (Mk 16:17). In his letters to the churches, the apostle Paul gave clear guidelines for dealing with the principalities and powers of this unseen world (Rom 1:18-23; 8:37; 1 Cor 10:20-22; Eph 1:20-23; 6:10-20; Col 1—2; 1 Tim 4:1-5; Jas 2:19).

Most people today—even many Christians—are biblically illiterate. With the loss of biblical knowledge in our culture, people do not know God or the spirit world as the Bible portrays them. Rationalist thinking taught us that we could know and conquer the natural world, using it for our purposes. Such thinking extended even to the social world, where we attempted to learn the laws that govern society, and to the inner world, where we mapped the psyche. Many of the social and psychological scientists early in the twentieth century had great hopes for remaking both human beings and society.

That quest for utopia clearly failed, with a resulting loss of faith in science. At the same time, Christianity has long been viewed as having been tried and found wanting; in fact, many modern problems are attributed to it by its critics. God, if he exists at all, is considered too far off to care about our problems; thus the return to pre-Christian religions (or new religions) with their rituals and occult practices.

Living in a Spiritual World

Even the church in the Western world has contributed to the problem of functional skepticism by not teaching and practicing the reality of God's daily involvement in our lives or the reality of eternal life. While people in difficult circumstances will talk of heaven, for many middle-class American Christians life here is good, and we want to keep it that way. We often think we don't need God to help us. After all, water comes out of the spigot when we turn it on. In more primitive cultures they pray for rain. If we are sick we take medicine or have surgery, and we pray as a last resort. However, even prayer is now being investigated scientifically. Christians, as well as skeptics and neopagans, are conducting research to see if prayer and other spiritual techniques work. Despite the postmodern disenchantment with science, we can't help thinking like modernists. We want to know how things work—and we want to control them.

Few Christians would overtly contradict the reality of the biblical worldview. But most of us function as if angels and demons were merely a vestige of primitive superstition. Many would go so far as to say that the Bible uses spiritual terminology to describe what we can now explain scientifically. For instance, in Mt 17:14-20 a man came to Jesus with his son who apparently was convulsing and falling into fires. In other records of this story (Mk 9:14-29; Lk 9:37-43) the father attributes the problem to a demon, but in this account he says the boy is "moonstruck" (from the Greek *selēniazetai*) or, as the KJV translates it, "a lunatic." Interestingly, newer translations struggle with this. The NIV is merely descriptive—the boy "has seizures"— but the NRSV and CEV come right out and diagnose the condition as "epilepsy." However, in all cases Jesus deals with the problem by rebuking "the demon," and the boy is cured.

While many in our culture today talk freely about angels and other supposedly benign spiritual forces, even many Christians do not acknowledge the reality of demons. Others see them behind every bush and live in fear. However, as nurses begin to flirt with the occult in therapeutic touch and other energy-based therapies, we believe that demonic activity will become much more evident. Both of us have seen evidence of this happening, in the United States as well as in other countries.

Arlene's Story

I (Arlene) lived in Zambia among people who were not only aware of spirits but sought to use and placate them. They attributed sickness and accidents to spirit activity. People who knew how to deal with spirits prescribed the rituals and formulas necessary to remove their evil influence. Unlike many Americans, who naively view spirits as helpful, these people feared them. Observing those under the influence of evil spirits was a terrifying experience. Two examples have stayed etched in my memory for many years.

One afternoon a woman was admitted to the hospital glassy-eyed and hyperventilating. She was brought from a local healer who dealt with spirits. Every woman in the forty-bed ward sat up as she was put in one of the beds. I sensed what they knew: this woman was under powerful spirit influence. Being an outsider to the culture, I wanted to confirm my impression with the hospital chaplain. After a bit of probing on my part, he agreed with my assessment, though indirectly. The word about this poor woman spread among patients, staff and nursing students.

The next morning I asked the students during our morning prayers if they wanted to pray for this woman. We had been reading in the Gospel of Mark about how Jesus delivered people from the power of evil spirits. I was a novice in such matters, but the issue seemed to be clearly before us. Many gathered at my home that evening and we prayed that Jesus would drive the evil spirit away. During the night the woman died! The next morning both I and the students were subdued. It seemed as if the Evil One had warned us to stay out of his territory. I decided that I would never try this again, at least not with such apparently difficult cases.

There were several times, however, when things went better. Once a young student complained for months of pain in one side of her body. Finally, after aspirin proved useless, I asked her what she thought the problem was. As I suspected, she thought that spirits were bothering her. She agreed to bring a friend with her to my office, and feeling somewhat foolish, I prayed she would be freed in Jesus' name. The pain went away! A short time later she was called home to attend a funeral. Because funerals involved rituals to drive spirits away, I feared that she might return to school with the old problem. But she did not, and never again did she come to the morning clinic complaining of pain in one side of her body.

Another story concerns a schoolteacher admitted to our hospital because she could not walk and refused to eat, a rather strange combination of symptoms. She had consulted but received no help from the local healer. Once again I sensed that spirit activity was part of the problem, but after the obvious failure with the woman who died, I resolved to stay uninvolved.

But one day, while supervising students in the unit, I watched this woman through the window in her room. She looked directly at me with eyes that I can only describe as burning. Surely there was help for this young woman. Since she was not eating, I wondered if she could be tempted with special foods.

She was! For some time I carried out a daily ritual of bringing her tasty food and trying to talk with her. She would not talk but slowly she began to walk. Finally, I gained sufficient courage to ask others to pray with me for her healing. We gathered around her, asking Jesus to drive out the spirit. She began to sing in a loud voice. Her mother, who had joined us, said that the spirit was singing. When she stopped singing we finished our prayer. She was not noticeably improved but continued to eat. After several weeks we transported her to the nearest psychiatric hospital, 180 miles away.

Undoubtedly this woman was psychotic, but spirits also were involved. I have thought that the combination of loving care, prayer for deliverance and psychiatric care were all part of her recovery.

Judy's Story

Early in my experience as a Nurses Christian Fellowship campus staff member, I (Judy) met with a new group of students. Ben, the group leader, told me beforehand that he was having difficulty leading Bible discussions and wanted help. As the meeting started, a strange phenomenon occurred. Whenever Ben would ask the group a question after reading a Bible passage, his face would contort. One side would be smiling and calm, the other side would scowl and twitch. The students on either side of him also responded in opposite ways. Those on the scowling side would sit in utter silence. Those on the smiling side would all talk at once.

After the meeting, Ben and I went for a walk to discuss what had happened. Ben was a good student and proud of his scientific objectivity, but finally he told me, "I think it's demons." As he spoke, his face contorted again, and his voice became uncharacteristically gruff. Surprised, I asked him what made him think so. He went on to tell me of a long family history of spiritualism. His grandmother regularly presided over seances in their dining room when he was a child. Before becoming a Christian he had consulted Ouija boards, smoked marijuana and often binged on alcohol. "I think I let evil spirits into my life. I know I'm a Christian, but there is still something that's not right," he confessed.

I knew nothing about demons then. My first inclination was to suggest he see a psychiatrist, but he replied that he had been in therapy for years. Finally, I talked with a colleague who had some experience with exorcism. He and another colleague met with Ben and cast out the demons. I was not present, but I could tell he was different. Ben experienced a radical change. From that point on he began to mature into a strong Christian leader. He never again suffered from his strange malady.

More recently I encountered the bizarre demonic world in a graduate course at a secular university. Trying to investigate the concepts being taught by the New Paradigm theorists, I enrolled in a course on "The Body—East and West." It was almost entirely East, after the West had been soundly maligned in the first three classes. The professor spoke freely of his own experiences in meditation, where he willingly entered the "demonic realm." He explained that during the early stages of meditation the demons would appear as serpents and monsters so frightening that "you could go crazy" without a spiritual advisor. However, in the later stages they would become "your friends." These friends often appeared to him as knights in shining armor and told him what to teach in class.

My classmates were almost all seekers or adherents of Eastern religions. Most were also practicing various forms of Eastern meditation as well as an eclectic assortment of spiritual exercises. I became increasingly uncomfortable in that class and began to literally shake as I drove home, so I desperately sought prayer support. My Sunday-school class and my husband prayed daily. Arlene would call me to pray over the phone before I left for class each week. With the prayer support I felt much more calm and confident, but the professor became much more aggressively anti-Christian. My class-mates, however, grew increasingly interested in knowing more about Chris-tianity.

One week we were to discuss the demonic realm in class. The readings had been horrible and vulgar. I enlisted more people to pray. When the professor came into the classroom that day, he walked over to me and bowed, which seemed strange to me and to several of my classmates sitting nearby. Then he told us that he couldn't teach what he had prepared for class because he "had a dream." He asked if anyone had any questions about the readings, but received only blank stares in return. Finally, he just started rambling on with a series of anti-Christian stories. I decided that this was not the time to retort, and so I sat calmly listening. Then he suddenly stopped and said, "I can't keep criticizing Christianity like this anymore, because Judy is going to get a gun and shoot me."

I laughed and said, "That wouldn't be very Christian!"

The woman to my left elbowed me and said, "That's his dream! He dreamed you shot him!"

But the ultimate test came when I turned in my final paper on the biblical view of the body (a topic he had approved). He gave it back to me and said, "You can't use this methodology. You've cited both the Old and New Testaments. You can't do that—those are two different gods. This is a B-paper unless you fix that." I did not "fix" it—but amazingly, I got an A- in the course.

Spirituality and Health Care

Although our experiences with the spirit world may seem bizarre and unconvincing, we can see strong parallels with the worldview expressed in the Scriptures. Western culture has been so strongly influenced by scientific "objectivity" that we have difficulty recognizing what people from the beginning of time have acknowledged and exploited.

People in almost every culture have developed various systems for relating to the spiritual realm, especially in regard to healing. Shamans—healers who gain their powers from the spirit world while in a trance-like state—have appeared indigenously on almost every continent. Attempts to appease malevolent spirits and attract familiar spirits through rituals and spiritual exercises are common around the world. Magicians try to compel gods, demons or spirits to do their bidding. They follow a pattern of occult practices to bend psychic forces to do their will. Even societies with atheistic philosophies, as well as those with strong monotheistic religions, including Christianity, have provided fertile soil for occult beliefs and practices. An undercurrent of paganism seems to lie dormant, even in Christianized cultures, only to resurface periodically. We are seeing just such a resurgence in many of the New Paradigm theories and therapies today.

Our primary concern in discussing spirituality is to look specifically at its relationship to health and health care. Probably the New Paradigm's greatest contribution to nursing is its strong emphasis on viewing the person holistically with a focus on the spiritual. However, as we have seen, spirituality cannot be generic or neutral. Energy-based therapies, prayer to other gods, or encouraging a person toward any spiritual beliefs and practices contrary to Christ only courts disaster. Even evidence that a particular alternative therapy appears to work does not necessarily make it permissible for the Christian nurse.

If we view Christian spirituality as the whole person in dynamic relationship with God through Jesus, then our definition impels us to nurture that relationship in contemplation, community and compassion for others. Rather than seeking a vague inwardness or manipulating of the spirit world, spirituality leads us to a mature faith and a life of service.

6

The Person
as a Cultural Being

A VISIBLY DISTRAUGHT MOTHER RUSHED INTO THE EMERgency room clutching a small child. Although the child appeared acutely ill, the mother spoke only Russian and could explain the problem only by making gestures. No one spoke Russian. Finally someone remembered the nurse on another unit who was also an Orthodox priest. When he arrived and spoke words of greeting in Russian, the mother calmed down. At last here was someone who would understand her plight. The physician diagnosed the child's illness, and treatment began.

As we have cared for people from other cultures in the course of our long nursing experience, we have seen all kinds of unusual practices—pans of water and pots of burning paper under beds, bags of herbs or amulets tied around necks, copper bracelets on arms and bottles of foul-smelling potions at the bedside—all purported to ward off various illnesses. Along the way we have learned some key words in other languages. Patients from various ethnic backgrounds and their families have enriched our nursing and introduced us to a wide variety of foods and customs.

Consider the following scene. I (Arlene) visited an African-American home in Pennsylvania with a Cambodian student. The grandmother was dying from congestive heart failure. The family had moved the living-room furniture into the dining room to make room for the grandmother's bed. While we were there, the pastor came to give communion. Then the grandson stopped in to see his parents and his grandmother. The dying woman's son was handicapped. The student and I were concerned about the weary daughter-in-law, who was the primary caregiver. It was a crowded, people-filled environment. Yet everyone present focused on the well-being of the dying woman.

My student from Cambodia, who was the only Christian in her Buddhist immigrant family, attempted to assess the needs of this multigenerational African-American family. My own Swiss-German heritage added another flavor to the mix, my father having been raised in the Amish church. I felt acutely aware of the cultural diversity. Yet we were joined in our common concern for the welfare of a dying woman.

Both of us (Arlene and Judy) have lived in other cultures outside the United States. We have been honored as guests in Asian, European and African homes. Returning this kindness to international guests has been our privilege. We have attended international conferences where nurses from many countries shared common concerns and also faced unique issues. The different cultural perspectives have broadened our thinking and enriched our lives.[1]

Most nursing texts today include information about cultural aspects of health and illness. Dr. Madeleine Leininger developed a nursing theory she calls Culture Care. In her book she relates the story of how she came to see the importance of educating nurses in cultural theory to improve nursing care.[2] Dr. Rachel Spector has spent years teaching and researching the rich cultural diversity in American society. Her book, *Cultural Diversity in Health and Illness*, first published in 1985, is now in its fourth edition. A literature search reveals a rapidly expanding body of material about cultural health practices in general nursing journals. Furthermore, a growing number of organizations and journals focuses entirely on cultural perspectives in nursing.[3]

The renewed interest in complementary, or alternative, health practices has exploded the interest in cultural health practices. Nursing and medical texts now include modalities from Native American, Chinese, Indian, Tibetan, Japanese, Latin American, African and pre-Christian European cultural traditions. In most instances these practices are presented as complementary to scientific medicine, not as replacements. Even though these texts present a plethora of practices, the common theme is that those using them must believe in them—the practices must be consistent with their larger belief system. The only criterion given for judging these practices from widely divergent cultures is whether or not they bring comfort and healing to the patient.

The diversity of human cultures shows many complex ways in which people have organized their social relationships and their response to their environment. The Bible itself reflects a diversity of cultures. Its writings were collected over a period of at least fifteen hundred years by people from a wide range of social backgrounds. "Customs are recorded from a diversity of middle-eastern, Judaic and Hellenistic cultures, though some are condemned, and none is regarded as ultimate."[4] Some people, whose stories we read in the Old Testament, thought that their culture reflected their life with God (Ruth, Samuel, Huldah), while others (Esther, Ezekiel, Daniel) were quite aware that their lives were lived over and against the dominant culture. "In the New Testament churches, no culture is identified as either wholly home for, or wholly inimical to, the gospel."[5]

Cultural Pluralism

Nurses are experiencing the cultural pluralism of our society and, even more, the cultural pluralism of the world. We are forced out of cultural isolation by modern communication and travel. We live in each other's neighborhoods: we see each other in health care settings. For the most part, we view this diversity as a positive development. Yet there is also trouble in the global village. Hatred between cultural and ethnic groups spills over into violence and war.

Our culture's conventional wisdom views tolerance as the virtue to resolve cultural conflict—tolerance for diversity in ideas and lifestyle. *Multiculturalism* is the widely used term describing North American society today—there are many cultures and subcultures. *Pluralism* and multiculturalism are related terms, describing the plurality of beliefs and practices in our world.

However, multiculturalism is only one aspect of pluralism. We encounter differing economic systems, political systems, philosophical systems and religions as well. Both of these concepts go beyond mere definition. Proponents tend to use them as political agendas for recognizing and respecting the differences within the human family. Furthermore, advocates of multiculturalism demand equal acceptance of all cultural viewpoints in academia and the workplace. Pluralism and multiculturalism, when used as philosophical or political positions, forego judgments about the relative goodness of any one culture. Tolerance, even approval, for all points of view and ways of living is advocated. Stan Gaede, however, asks the question, "Is tolerance based on a commitment to truth and justice, or is it merely indifference?"[6] We will return to this question later.

A Christian Understanding of Culture

What do we mean by culture? There are numerous definitions, and none of them is completely adequate. Some are so broad as to include the total way of life of a group of people. Others are very abstract—for example, culture as a set of symbols. Missionary theologian Bruce Nicholls defines culture as "the sum total of the learned behavior patterns and attitudes of a given community."[7] His thinking guides much of our discussion about culture.

Culture is learned, passed on from one generation to another through a process of *enculturation*. It is the *nurture*, not *nature*, aspect of human behavior. Enculturation is both deliberate and conscious, when we are taught by parents, teachers and clergy. Yet it also happens unconsciously, when we imitate elders and peers and absorb their values and ideas. Because culture is acquired, not inherited, it is constantly changing—sometimes rapidly and at other times more slowly. Even traditional cultures that are not exposed to outside influences change.

Several models help us to understand the various aspects of culture and how they relate to one another. One model pictures culture as a series of four layers.[8] The deepest layer consists of the cultural worldview, assumptions that answer questions about people and the world: (1) What is prime reality—the really real? (2) What is the nature of external reality, the world around us? (3) What is a human being? (4) What happens to a person at death? (5) How is it possible to know anything at all? (6) How do we know what is right and wrong? (7) What is the meaning of human history?[9] The second layer, closely related and largely derived from the worldview, is that of values, particularly ethical and moral values. Based on both the worldview and values, the next layer of culture is social institutions such as marriage, law, education and so on. Finally, at the surface but growing out of the layers below, there is the layer of material artifacts (technology, art, clothing) and observable behavior and customs. This surface layer is more easily described and more easily changed. It is this layer where nurses see health-related practices. (See figure 3.)

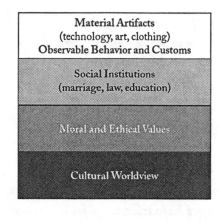

Figure 3. Levels of culture

Nicholls suggests that the interaction between these layers of a culture can be viewed as a pyramid with the worldview as an unseen hidden base. The values, institutions and observable behavior form the three sides interacting with each other. (See figure 4.)

Anthropologists consider religion integral to culture—a *human factor* influencing and influenced by each aspect of the culture. *Religion* is a slippery term and hard to define. It can be applied to the assumptions of a worldview, even if the culture claims to be secular, because worldviews are based on faith, not empirical observations. Secular societies relegate religious practices to people's private lives. In more religious societies, such as tribal groups and some Islamic countries, religion permeates all levels of the culture and strongly influences health practices. Anthropologists focus their study on the human side of religion.

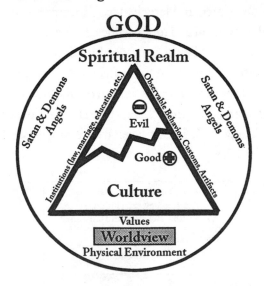

Figure 4.   Culture and worldview

The Supracultural Realm

From a Christian perspective, religion is far more than a human factor. Throughout this book we have referred to reality as both seen and unseen. Nicholls refers to unseen reality as the *supracultural realm*—"the phenomena of cultural belief and behavior that have their source outside of human culture."[10] The biblical writers assume the reality of a spiritual realm which includes God, angels, Satan and demons. In contrast, secular anthropologists assume that all the factors that determine religion are contained within the culture itself. Christians accept the biblical view that the unseen reality—the supracultural realm—interacts with the culture.

God works in human history to establish his rule in the hearts of those who accept the gospel. The church is the community of those who have come under his rule. "It follows therefore, that where Christ is truly Lord of his church the cultural design for living of its members will be different from those of the wider community. There will be a progressive movement toward a 'Christian culture' which will reflect both the universality of the gospel and the particularity of the human environment."[11] For example, the fruit of the Holy Spirit will be present in a church of a particular culture, as in Christian churches elsewhere. At the same time, each church will reflect the specific culture of which it is a part, but to some extent divested of the worldview, values and customs that are contrary to the gospel.[12]

We see many examples where Christians are different from and yet identify with their larger culture. Navajo Christians retain the strong Navajo sense of family and their keen awareness of the spirit world. Instead of calling the hand-trembler and medicine man for the traditional healing "sing," they substitute Christian prayer at community camp meetings. Zambian Christians reject the traditional practice of polygamy and teach monogamous marriage instead. But they retain the culture's concern for support and help within the extended family. In North America, Christians struggle to free themselves from the rampant individualism of our culture and yet retain a strong sense of personal responsibility. Korean Christians maintain their deep respect for the elderly. At the same time they gather for daily early-morning prayer meetings instead of practicing traditional shamanistic rituals.

The boundary line between what is Christian and what belongs to the culture can be exceedingly difficult to draw. Only Christ's lordship and the illumination of the Holy Spirit on Scripture can guide the individual Christian and the church to make this distinction. It is usually best done by those within the culture itself, rather than by outsiders. At the same time those from other cultures often see things about beliefs and practices to which insiders are blind. For example, African and Asian Christians help North Americans to see the way we neglect our elders. Christians from poor countries help us to see how often we equate God's blessing with affluence.

The *demonic* comprises the other supracultural source of cultural beliefs and practices. As we saw earlier, Satan is a powerful spiritual being ruling over other evil beings. Satan is a real being whom John calls "the ruler of this world" (Jn 12:31; 14:30; 16:11). John also says that "the whole world lies under the power of the evil one" (1 Jn 5:19). Paul writes of Satan seducing people to worship him (1 Cor 15:24, 26; Eph 1:21; 3:10; 6:12; Col 1:16; 2:10, 15). The world is not a closed system, as secular anthropologists believe; it is the arena of a battle between the kingdom of God and the kingdom of Satan.[13] Although Christ decisively won the victory over Satan on the cross, it is being worked out in human history. The culmination will come with the return of Christ to establish his reign on earth. In the meantime the effects of the conflict are played out within every culture. Look again at figure 4, where the chasm between good and evil runs right through the culture. No culture is fully good or completely evil.

And culture is never neutral. Each culture contains evidence of both of evil and of God's goodness. On one occasion, when Paul and Barnabas healed a man in Jesus' name, the crowd wanted to worship them. The people thought these men were appearances of the gods Zeus and Hermes, and the priest was prepared to sacrifice to them. Paul and Barnabas barely restrained them with these words:

> Friends, why are you doing this? We are mortals just like you, and we are bringing you good news, that you should turn from these worthless things to the living God, who made the heaven and the earth and the sea and all that is in them. In the past generations he allowed all the nations to follow their own ways; *yet he has not left himself without a witness in doing good—giving you rains from heaven and fruitful seasons, and filling you with food and your hearts with joy* (Acts 14:15-17, italics ours).

Both good and evil were present in that culture just as they are in every other culture, including our own.

Recognizing the supracultural source of evil explains the similarities of evil in many different cultures. Eugene D. Dukes compares the practice of modern witchcraft with medieval witchcraft. He concludes: "It certainly is placing a heavy burden on the reader and student to accept as coincidence or misinterpretation the closeness in appearance of modern witchcraft as now practiced with the medieval variety. I think it is obviously true *that a single source of supernatural evil best explains this similarity*" (italics ours).[14]

We would extend this conclusion to other kinds of evil in both ancient and modern cultures. One example is the widespread abuse of women, of which female genital mutilation is a prime example. Another example is trying to manipulate the natural world through rituals, mental techniques and shamanistic trances. These practices have similar characteristics whether in the religions condemned by the ancient Hebrew prophets or the current "new religions" and reversions to pre-Christian religions.

Likewise, God manifests his goodness in similar ways in every culture. Human beings bear God's image, both as individuals and as a social group. The gift of language enables people to create culture and to pass on traditions. All cultures have some idea of the family as the foundation for social organization. All cultures have respect for human life. All persons show God's gift of creativity when they create institutions, art and music—all things beautiful. At the same time, because of human rebellion against the Creator, humans look to their own creations to save them. Paul wrote: "They exchanged the truth about God for a lie and worshiped and served the creature rather than the Creator" (Rom 1:25). This is the essence of idolatry.

"Idolatry is the worst sin of all, because it moves God to the periphery of our lives and puts something else in his place."[15] In the eighth century B.C. the prophet Isaiah railed against the idolatry of the Hebrews, the very people God had chosen for his own (Is 44:6-23). Idolatry is not only offensive to God, it is absurd; those who feed on it feed on ashes and their deluded hearts deceive them (v. 20). Human beings make idols (v. 9) but the Lord has made Israel [the Hebrews] (v. 21) and displays his glory through her (v. 23). What an honor![16] Likewise, those in God's kingdom are to bring honor to him. Jesus said to his followers, "You are the light of the world. A city built on a hill cannot be hid. . . . Let your light shine before others, so that they may see your good works and give glory to your Father in heaven" (Mt 5:14, 16).

The danger of idolatry, in one enticing form or another, is always with us. "Chameleon-like, it constantly disguises itself so that we are scarcely aware of its presence, even when we are most in the grip of it."[17] The apostle Paul writes that greed is idolatry, because it puts things in place of God, looking to them to bring satisfaction and salvation (Col 3:5). Cruder forms of idolatry, such as worshiping images of gods, may seem far removed from secular Americans. Yet looking to crystals (things God created) to bring spiritual healing, wearing amulets (bags of herbs or objects of art) to protect us from evil or using mental techniques (various forms of energy manipulation) are no less idolatry. They all are seeking from other sources what only God can do for us.

Jesus Christ, the Only Way to God

In the present climate of cultural pluralism, saying that the biblical worldview is correct and that Jesus is the only way to God offends many. How can all other religions be wrong? We do not claim that *everything* taught and practiced in other religions is wrong. There are some true aspects of other religions. For example, they may be understood as expressions of the longings for communion with God, an essential human characteristic. We were created to worship and serve him.[18] An example of this longing is the Temple of Heaven, in Beijing, where the emperor offered yearly sacrifices for the blessings of heaven. The architecture of the circular buildings is beautiful, and the many altars with plaster images of sacrificial cattle surrounding the main temple speak of human awareness of the need for sacrifice.

Yet even though traces of truth and beauty can be seen in other religions, Christians believe "there is salvation in no one else, for there is no other name under heaven given among mortals by which we must be saved" (Acts 4:12). While such a claim is indeed exclusive, we would note that, when taken seriously, all other religions are also exclusive. Those who argue that all religions are the same, or that they are only different paths to the same God, have only a superficial understanding of what each of them teaches. Each religion prescribes a path of salvation, and each one describes a different god or gods. To argue this point is beyond the focus of this chapter. We only want to say that it is the very nature of religion to make exclusive claims. So we make no apology for the exclusive claims of Christianity.

At the same time, Christianity is the most inclusive of religions. Many other religions are ethnic in nature, including only those of a certain tribe or race. Christianity encompasses people worldwide in every culture. Even the Old Testament, in which God specifically chooses the Jews as his special people, alludes to this international character of God's kingdom. God called

Abraham from the city of Ur with its pagan religion to follow him—in other words, Abraham had to change his religion.

God promised Abraham that all the nations of the earth would be blessed through him and his descendants (Gen 18:8). The apostle Paul wrote that this promise was fulfilled in Jesus Christ (Gal 3:14). God spoke through the Hebrew prophet Zechariah: "Many nations shall join themselves to the Lord on that day, and shall be my people; and I will dwell in your midst" (Zech 2:11). Jesus' last words to his disciples instructed them to proclaim the good news to all nations: "Go therefore and make disciples of all nations, baptizing them in the name of the Father and of the Son and of the Holy Spirit, and teaching them to obey everything that I have commanded you" (Mt 28:19-20). John, to whom God gave a vision of the new heaven and earth, wrote that in the heavenly city, lighted by God's glory:

> The nations will walk by its light, and the kings of the earth will bring their glory into it. . . . People will bring into it the glory and the honor of the nations. But nothing unclean will enter it, nor anyone who practices abomination or falsehood, but only those who are written in the Lamb's book of life (Rev 21:24, 26-27).

God both judges and redeems all cultures with their religions. What is evil must be put away; what is good will be transformed and preserved. God extends his grace to all through the work of Jesus Christ—his death and resurrection. The apostle Paul wrote, "May I never boast of anything except the cross of the Lord Jesus Christ, by which the world has been crucified to me, and I to the world" (Gal 6:14).

Nursing, Health and Culture

In light of both the exclusiveness and the inclusiveness of God's invitation in Jesus Christ, we turn to those observable aspects of culture where nurses practice. Nursing texts are replete with lists of how culture affects health care. Rachel Spector cites six categories: environmental control, biological variations, social organization, communication, space, and time orientation.[19] Most texts include discussions about cultural views of birth, health, illness, death and behaviors associated with each of these. There is usually some discussion of various folk remedies and healing practices. True to the multicultural emphasis of our own culture and of nursing, these practices are usually described with no attempt to evaluate them other than how they might benefit the patient's sense of well-being or recovery.

Health-related practices belong to the most superficial level of observable behavior in a culture. At the same time, most nurses in secular North America have not been accustomed to considering the relationship between folk practices and the underlying worldview. The worldview and religious links of such practices may not be explicit. However, more writers are beginning to identify these underlying cultural views and links with approval.[20]

Problems of Cultural Relativism

One problem with cultural and religious pluralism is that *human salvation* becomes the heart and norm of all religion, "thereby making the human self the decisive center of all meaning and value. Such pluralism is egocentric and fundamentally similar to monistic religions such as Hinduism and the New Age philosophy."[21] Following this approach to health care is not an option for Christians. Making *health* the sole criterion for evaluating a practice is misguided.[22] Bringing honor to God's name by obeying him is what should guide us.

First we must ask how various health practices, with their worldview and religious underpinnings, promote God's honor. Even though these practices represent the most superficial layer of a culture, their worldview and religious links must be discerned because they may have serious implications and effects. A leading nurse-advocate of alternative therapies says these "healing rituals both reflect and create the values of an individual and a culture."[23]

In other words, health-related practices create values and worldviews as well as reflect them. This is true whether the practices are shamanistic or scientific and high-tech. Rather than giving uncritical acceptance to a different worldview, we must use critical judgment when assessing health-related practices. For example, many persons who were originally skeptical of therapeutic touch have been convinced by what they experienced and subsequently changed their view of life.[24]

Observable behavior and the underlying worldview and values (the area of religion) can be separated. Sometimes people do the right thing for the wrong reason. For example, some forms of massage are based on the theory that it balances the flow of *chi*. However, the benefits of massage can be explained physiologically through processes of muscle relaxation and blood flow. For centuries people learned those things that promote health through trial and error, long before they could explain them scientifically. Much of even present-day health care practice remains empirical; we know it seems to work but not exactly how and why. The scientific fields of psychoneuroimmunology (PNI) and psychoneuroendocrinology (PNE) have described many of the physiological responses associated with psychological states. Neither PNI or PNE, however, can establish the exact mechanism between states of mind and the bodily response.

If some alternative therapies seem to relieve pain or help patients relax, it seems best to admit that we just do not know how they work, rather than to explain them in a way that conflicts with Scripture. Some practices, however, require that the users suspend judgment based on their own religious beliefs in order for the method to work. Some go even further and advocate entering into the unseen reality, or *supracultural realm,* through meditative techniques that put the meditator in contact with spiritual beings. Such practices bypass the clear scriptural teaching that we can approach God only through Jesus Christ.

In some practices the ties to specific religions and worldviews are so close that it is not possible for followers of Jesus to use these therapies.[25] Other practices—massage or use of herbs, for example—can be separated from non-Christian roots.[26] Well-designed research may help us find a physiological explanation, and then again we may need to rely on empirics.

Other Problems of Multiculturalism

Beyond the religious worldview problems of multiculturalism, other problems related to pluralism and multiculturalism are being raised by nurses. June F. Kikuchi, Helen Simmons and Donna Romyn sound an alarm for nurses who are increasingly accepting a subjective view of reality.[27] They are concerned about *epistemology*—how and what we can know about reality. If there really is no objective reality and everything that exists is only an individual or cultural perception, then how can nurses agree on what is true about nursing? How can nurses from different cultures come to any agreement about standards for nursing? If every worldview is equally acceptable, can we even communicate with each other? Is there a way to think about reality—our environment—that allows for both diversity and universality? Of course, we believe that the biblical worldview does exactly this.

June Kikuchi also sees multicultural ethics as a potential threat to responsible nursing practice. She takes issue with advocates of multicultural ethics who claim that diversity is the only thing to say about human behavior—that people have nothing in common beyond physiological functioning. In other words, there is no such thing as human nature. She also argues against multiculturalists who deny the possibility of deriving any universal, objective moral truths from experience. She explores the implications of saying that moral conduct can be guided and judged only by the values and norms of each particular culture, that any claims for universal moral principles are false. She concludes that this view, taken to its logical conclusion, would prevent nurses from trying to influence or change the health practices of anyone from another culture than their own.

In practice, nurses who say that ethical teachings are entirely subjective and relative to each culture violate their own beliefs when they try to influence the behavior of members of another culture. She gives the example of a nurse trying to change the minds of parents who are refusing immunizations for their children because of religious beliefs.

Kikuchi is correct in her concern for the implications of multicultural ethics. Readers who have followed us so far in this book will know that we (Arlene and Judy) do believe there is a common human nature beyond the physical. Further, God has shown us what is good, what should guide our ethics. We can observe human life to gain moral knowledge, as Kikuchi suggests. But more than that, God has given us, in Scripture, guidelines that shed light on our experience. We are not left to human reason alone to discern moral principles.

Guidelines for Finding Our Way

After the preceding discussion, we are ready for some practical guidelines for finding our way in a culturally pluralistic world. Theologian Charles Sherlock suggests three general approaches:

1. We should put away the idea that any one culture embodies Christian faith (this is especially true for those of us who live in cultures that have been most influenced by Christianity).

2. We should use crosscultural relationships to reflect on our own culture—both to identify our prejudices and to be enriched by others' experiences and ways of thinking.

3. We must recognize the effects of sin on all human cultures: the outworkings of human pride, self-centeredness and the desire to be in control are present in every culture.[28]

We also return to the question raised early in this chapter, "Is tolerance based on commitment to justice and truth or is it merely indifference?" We can respond that there is a kind of tolerance based on commitment to the God of truth and justice, who respects the freedom of every person to choose either to follow him or to reject his ways. Those who reject him, however, will find themselves in bondage to evil that leads ultimately to spiritual death. But this same God is also the God of love, who invites, even pleads with his creatures to return to him. He is not indifferent; he acts with sacrificial love.

What does this kind of tolerance look like for Christian nurses? Here are some guidelines for nursing in a pluralistic world:

Avoid ethnocentrism. Judging other cultures by the standards of our own is wrong. Scripture, rightly interpreted, is the only standard by which cultures are to be judged.

Beware of radical cultural relativism. The view that truth, ethics and standards for health care can be defined only from within each specific culture is not a valid position. There *are* transcultural truths, ethics and standards for nursing. Nurses should work to define these in intercultural conferences and research.

Practice modified cultural relativism. Appreciation for the many cultural practices that make sense only within specific cultures is the best approach. It brings joy, and often frustration, to crosscultural relationships. Taking off one's shoes makes a lot of sense in Korean homes where traditionally people sit on the floor to eat and roll out mats for sleeping. We can learn much from the health practices of other cultures. Congenital hip displacement in children is not seen in rural Zambia. Infants may have been born with shallow acetabulums, but the way mothers carry them on their backs for two years provides a natural corrective splint.

Remember that humility and toleration are essential virtues. Humility will keep us from being closed-minded about what seems negative in others' ways of doing things. Much of what seems senseless or wrong is simply our misunderstanding. We begin by learning, observing, inquiring and trying to understand. Tolerance will help us to love in spite of differences that annoy or offend. It is a tolerance based not on indifference but on commitment to God's honor and his grace extended both to us and to others.

Accept people where they are. God takes a long time to work out his purposes in our lives. This is true both as individuals and within a culture. Practice kindness and courtesy even when health practices are clearly in conflict with the scriptural teaching. If the person is a Christian, you can give reasons for why you think the practice is wrong and then trust the Holy Spirit to convince the person in his time. If the person is of another religion or says he or she has no religion, you can simply explain that you see things differently because you are a Christian.

Remember that the freedom to make choices—and accept the consequences— reflects God's image in us. Letting people make decisions about their own health care is not the same as condoning what they are doing.

Communicate in ways that are easily understood. Learning the language of those among whom we work is the highest form of respect. Having culturally appropriate literature is essential. Do those things that bring comfort and security to patients and families, even if they seem senseless to you, as long as they are not actually harmful to their health.

Refrain from practices and techniques that are clearly prohibited for Christians. Those customs connected to nonbiblical worldviews or non-Christian religions can be tied to evil powers. If rituals involve spirits, angels, demons, gods or goddesses, Christian should not be involved. Sometimes, in order to learn, observing such rituals and practices may be helpful, but not actual participation.

Pray, first, last and always. Ask God for wisdom, for understanding, for discernment. Pray that the Holy Spirit will work through you to make God's truth and love real in the situation. Pray for an opening to talk about Jesus Christ.

An Example of Crosscultural Nursing

Sonia, a friend of ours who works in India, exemplifies the best in crosscultural nursing. One of her patients was an elderly Sikh gentleman who was dying. She went out of her way to give him excellent care and in so doing endeared herself to his family. When the man died, the family asked her to take part in the funeral services. She agreed—and prayed for wisdom as to how she should participate in the ceremonies. After arriving she asked the Sikh priest if she would be permitted to sing a Christian hymn. He agreed, and when the time came she stood and sang. While singing she noticed tears in the eyes of the priest.

I (Arlene) asked her what she would do if a dying Hindu patient wanted her to chant prayers to Shiva, a common Hindu practice with dying patients. She replied that she could not do that, but she often asked for permission to pray to her God until the Hindu priest arrived. Patients rarely refused. She would send for the patient's religious leader if she was requested to do so. She prays for wisdom in her nursing interventions, guided by knowledge of Scripture and trusting the Holy Spirit to lead her. She models the meaning of Christian crosscultural nursing.

Part Three

The Environmental Context for Nursing

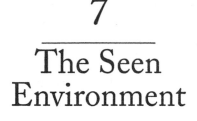

7

The Seen Environment

AFTER YEARS OF HOSPITAL NURSING, LIZ STARTED TO WORK in a rural home health agency covering eight counties. The tenuous living situation of many patients was nearly overwhelming at first. She prayed for guidance to know which of her patients needed special attention. One family—a mother and stepson—was particularly troublesome. The eighty-four-year-old woman was dependent upon her stepson for much of her care. The obese son was himself confined to a wheelchair. Even though the nursing care was simple enough, the dirty, foul-smelling house was repugnant. In spite of that, Liz discovered two likable people, discouraged about their situation but doing the best they could.

As Christmas approached Liz decided that it was time to do something extra. She doubted that there would be any Christmas at this home. One afternoon, she went loaded with a small tree, decorations, Christmas cookies and a few small gifts. The mother and son were overwhelmed! Tears flowed. Liz learned much that afternoon about the past life of this woman who had survived some very difficult times. She began to pray earnestly for them and wondered how to tell them of God's love for them.

Some time later Liz and a friend spent an afternoon there helping with cleaning and laundry. Much trash was bagged to be taken away. Because there was no washer in the home, Liz took several loads of laundry with her. As she lay in bed that evening she thought about this family, so needy and yet trying to maintain some dignity. She thought of others in her case load, many of them angry, frightened or lonely people. "God," she prayed, "you have put these people in my life. You love them and know their needs. Let me be your hands for them."

The Environment in Nursing

Modern public health nursing was born in the optimistic glow of late nineteenth- and early twentieth-century science. Florence Nightingale's promotion of district nursing, distinct from sick nursing, was her vision for improving the general health of the British population.[1] Her *Notes on Nursing*, written for every woman who had charge of the health of others, focused on the immediate environment of the ill person. Nightingale believed that controlling the environment "put the patient in the best possible condition" for nature to do its healing. Discovering the laws of nature would enable us to do this.[2] District nursing brought this knowledge to the homes of the average person. Early American public health nursing was directed toward teaching people how to live in a healthy way. In many ways these efforts were successful: parents had their infants vaccinated, schoolchildren learned about healthy diets, pregnant women attended prenatal clinics, people learned first aid to care for injuries and wounds.

Yet a committee appointed by the National Institute for Medicine recently reported that nurses need better preparation to deal with stubborn environmental health issues.[3] The committee defined *environmental health* as "freedom from illness or injury related to exposure to toxic agents and other environmental conditions that are potentially detrimental to human health." The environmental hazards addressed by the committee fell into four classes: chemical, physical, biological and psychosocial.[4] There was general agreement about addressing the health problems in these areas. Yet the committee noted that there is "heated debate over others that exist between health and social problems," such as interpersonal violence.[5] A great number of the problems encountering public health nurses fall into this contested area of social causes of disease. We will consider it in the next chapter.

Some health care workers, in reaction to failures of modern medicine, have turned to another solution. A popular magazine recently carried a photo of Andrew Weil, a physician advocate of natural holistic healing therapies, covered with mud and sporting a green herb.[6] The picture is symbolic of those who see the hope for health in a return to the unspoiled world of nature. Decrying the failures of aggressive scientific medicine and technology, they offer a bewildering menu of therapies ranging from herbs to energy manipulation to shamanistic rituals to mystical channeling of ancient spirit beings. In contrast to those in the public health movement who promote controlling the physical and social environment through public policy, these advocates of "natural healing" by and large eschew government regulation in health issues. They advocate instead a kind of do-it-yourself approach. Rather than controlling the environment, their philosophy is one of merging with or finding harmony with it.

Much of current nursing literature on the environment has similar themes. One nurse educator describes her understanding of the environment as "alive, whole and interacting," reflected in the Gaia hypothesis, which states that the world is "a system made up of all living things and their environment. There is no clear distinction, only graded intensities, between living and non-living matter."[7] She looks to the ideas of the ancient Greeks and Romans and traditional Native Americans, as well as Eastern philosophy, for her understanding of the environment. She eventually concludes that the entire planet is our nursing client.[8]

For some nurses this language of merging takes on religious overtones:

> We must rejoin ourselves, individually and collectively, with a caring consciousness, a living cosmology that unites and attunes scientific forces with the myth, mystery, and metaphor of the mythic and mystical forces that reside on the other side of the universe that is continually turning over.
>
> The last step is crossing over the internal bridge of our consciousness and entering into this *living caring cosmology for our Lost Mother*.[9]

Both the public health approach and the merging approach are based on certain assumptions about the world around us, about the environment and about the larger reality in which we live. The public health approach reflects the modern paradigm of science and reason in which the goal is to control the environment, including people if need be, in order to eradicate disease. The second approach of merging and harmony with the environment is characteristic of the New Paradigm to which many thinkers in nursing are turning.

Early theories were primarily concerned with the patient's immediate physical environment or, in the case of community health, the larger environment including housing, transportation, food, water and so on. Today many include the social environment as well. Some include the whole earth and even the universe. Martha Rogers removed time boundaries past and present in the environment.[10]

What does the Christian worldview tell us about our human dwelling? In the remainder of this chapter we will consider the seen environment, the natural world. In the next chapter we will turn to the unseen spiritual environment and its influence on our social relationships.

The Meaning of Natural

What do we mean when we refer to the natural environment? It is important to be clear about this because the term *natural* has taken on many connotations today. We are referring to the world of physical (material) things, those aspects of creation studied by natural science: biology, chemistry, physics and all their various branches. The natural world is the carbon-based dimension in which we live.

Natural has become a code word today representing opposition to excessive use of technology, a "back to nature" approach similar to the "merging with nature" view discussed earlier. Natural foods are raised without commercial fertilizers. Natural childbirth is delivery without use of anesthetics, most often by midwives. Herbal medicine is preferred over synthetic, manufactured drugs. Naturopathic medicine, a movement of the early 1900s, is reemerging. Naturopathy asserts "the healing power of nature" and focuses on nutrition, lifestyle and environment.[11]

When Florence Nightingale spelled *nature* with a capital *N*, she was close to if not totally endorsing this view. From a Christian perspective there may be much that is right about some of these approaches. On the other hand, embedded in the explanations there are often assumptions about nature that are not supported by Scripture.

Does nature have the power to heal? Yes and no. If we mean by this that God has built into our bodies processes that destroy invading organisms and restore damaged tissues, the answer is yes. The immune system and processes of tissue regeneration belong to the natural world. They are not wise and benevolent in themselves; such attributes belong only to the Creator.[12] Natural processes are simply working as their Creator designed them. Nursing interventions support these natural processes: dressing changes to remove drainage, exercises for cardiovascular and muscular strengthening, rest to conserve energy, nutrition to sustain the immune system and tissue repair, bathing and turning to prevent skin breakdown, teaching healthy lifestyles. As we do these things we are fulfilling God's intention that we care for and develop the natural world.

Does nature have power to heal? If by that we mean that the body has consciousness and intention in itself for healing should be left to itself, then the answer is no—nature does not heal. Nature is not a wise and benevolent physician. It has no conscious intentions of its own. Only God, who created the natural world, is wise and has good intentions for creation.[13] As we saw above, God has given humankind the responsibility to carry out his intentions. Nursing is one way of doing so.

Another Question About Nature

A question concerning many in nursing today, especially when confronted with claims of alternative therapies, is, What is the ultimate "stuff" of the natural world? Nurses are acquainted with molecules and atoms. Most of us know something of the debate concerning light: does light consist of particles or waves, or both? We hear the terms *quantum physics, Heisenberg uncertainty principle* and *field theory*. But we may fail to see the meaning of much of this for nursing. It seems sufficient to understand molecular functions in fluid and electrolyte balance and pharmacology, and radioactivity in radiation-based diagnosis and therapy. We are glad to benefit from research on viruses done with the electron microscope and from new treatments based on subatomic theories. Meanwhile we give our attention to caring for people.

Now, however, we are being asked to learn a new language about energy. The addition in 1994 of *energy field disturbance* to the NANDA listing of nursing diagnoses is an example.[14] What does this mean?

The concept of energy has long been familiar to nurses. We understand that metabolism releases energy for body functioning and work. We know that oxygen is required for metabolism and for the functioning of all body systems. We know about electrons in the electrical functions of the heart, brain and muscles. We also know something about radioactivity—its use in diagnosis and treatment and its potential for harm. Some of us may know about field theories in physics. But what is the human energy field theory?

Martha Rogers introduced this concept of energy field to nursing. Using the language of physics, she described people and their environment as energy fields. It is important to note that in her view humans do not *have* or *generate* energy fields; they *are* energy fields. She meant something other than the electrical activity of muscles and nerves creating an energy field around a person; instead, being human equaled being an energy field. Failed early attempts at New York University, where Rogers was Dean of the School of Nursing, to measure human energy fields were first explained by lack of sensitive instrumentation. Since then explanations tend to focus on a unique energy not accessible to physical measurement.

Many nurses who followed Rogers's thinking abandoned the idea that physics itself supported what they meant by *human energy field*. They appropriated various ideas, many from the Eastern philosophies and religions.[15] Nurses began reading of *qi, chi, ki, prana,* and *vital* or *life force* as explanations for therapies based on human field theory. Translated as "energy," these terms all convey the notion that there is a life-giving energy flowing through the universe, through the earth and through all living beings. Health results from balance and movement in this energy, illness from blockage or depletion. Techniques to restore the balance and flow of energy vary from hand movements to directing of mental intentions toward individuals or situations. Food, exercise and meditation are also used to restore the energy balance.

Because these energies, sometimes called *subtle energy*, cannot be measured directly, research has focused on their supposed effects: increased positive affect, decreased negative affect, pain relief and sense of relaxation.

Still the modern reliance on physics dies hard, and many writers explain these effects by referring to quantum physics and electromagnetism. It is doubtful whether most of those relying on such explanations understand quantum theory. Yet this "quantum leap" in thinking is frequent in nursing literature. Using the language of science lends an aura of respectability to human energy-field theory and the interventions based upon it. Advocates go even farther when they elevate energy field to the level of worldview.

Quantum mechanics does not apply to the world of people and things in which nurses work.[16] There is no evidence based on physics that "intention" alone, so central to energy-based theories, brings about changes either in the physiology of other persons or in the environment. Even if we limit the changes in our patients brought about by a nurse's intention to psychological or social changes, some communication, either verbal or non-verbal, must occur. Thoughts in the nurse's mind must be acted upon in order to bring about changes in another person.

The human brain is part of the seen world; the human mind belongs to the unseen world. The two are related and influence one another, yet they are distinct. Philosophers and scientists have debated the "mind-body" problem for years with no cause-and-effect explanation for how they do interact. But those who have elevated notions of nuclear physics to a worldview argue that brain and mind are fundamentally the same. Not willing to yield to a mechanical view of things, they see the environment as a giant conscious system encompassing all reality. (Others argue for some higher reality that is neither matter nor consciousness.)[17] All things—rocks, earth, cells—are seen as conscious, with innate powers of consciousness and healing. There is no mind/body separation in this view, for all is mind. Phenomena like *nonlocal* healing are explained by the ability of thought (alone) to influence far-distant events. Advocates claim to have reduced the amount of crime in a city when many people meditate at the same time.[18]

Clearly they have left the science of physics and have embarked on philosophy.

Brilliant physicists continue to speculate about the fundamental nature of things. However, when matter is subdivided to its absolute smallest level, whether particles, waves or energy, the next thing is nothing physical and we *must* turn to either philosophy or theology. Eastern religions have elevated nothing to the *Nothing* or the *Void*, as ultimate reality. In the biblical worldview something does exist beyond the smallest possible division of matter—the personal God of the Bible. This is the God who creates out of nothing and who sustains all things by his word. God is the ultimate source of the life and energy sought by those using the human-energy theory. God is also the Creator of the whole continuum of motion, from quantum mechanics of the smallest particles to classical mechanics of the familiar world of things and people in which nurses work.

There are distinctions between kinds of created things in this world. The Genesis story of creation supports this idea. "Thus the heavens and the earth were finished, and all their multitude" (Gen 2:1). God had different kinds of things in mind when he created them. The concept of species is implied in the Hebrew word *min* that describes the reproduction of plants and animals in the Creation story. God made clear distinctions between the kinds of animals the Hebrews could eat (Gen 1:1-25; Lev 11:14-29). Even though God made many kinds of things from the same basic physical "stuff," their uniqueness and distinctiveness remains. Rather than turning to Nothing or the Void to find harmony and unity, we turn to God, the Creator.

We (Arlene and Judy) have had many conversations with believers in *chi*, both from cultures where this idea has a long tradition and from "new believers" in Western countries, about what this energy is. Could it reflect a longing for the tree of life from which Adam and Eve were banned after their sin? Could it be an attempt to gain life in a way that God has not made available to us, life that only he will restore when the time is right? It's an understanding that may help to explain why similar ideas are found in so many cultures and religions. The good news is that God will give us the eternal life for which we were created and for which we long. But the Bible makes it clear that he does that only through Jesus Christ.

The Natural Creation Gives Us Clues About God

The first thing to say about our environment, then, is that it is the creation of a personal, loving Creator. All created things, living and nonliving, are dependent on him for their existence. At the same time the created environment is distinct from God the Creator. This is quite different from saying "Matter is all there is and all there ever was," as is assumed in the modern scientific worldview. It is also quite different from assuming the existence of an impersonal *chi* (breath or vital force) as the source of life.[19] Nor is this the same thing as viewing all reality as god or the earth as our Mother. While creation is dependent upon God, God is not dependent for his being upon creation. In other words, the creation is not God.

However, while creation is not a manifestation of God, it does express much of what God is like, just as a work of art reveals much about the artist. The psalmist writes:

> The heavens are telling the glory of God;
>   and the firmament proclaims his handiwork.
> Day to day pours forth speech,
>   and night to night declares knowledge.
> There is no speech, nor are there words;
>   their voice is not heard;
> yet their voice goes out through all the earth,
>   and their words to the end of the world.
>   (Ps 19:1-4)

Observing the natural world tells us that God is powerful, that he is wise and that he provides for his creation. Psalm 104 gives us a picture of all creatures rejoicing in dependence on God's creative and gracious power:

> These all look to you
>   to give them their food in due season;
> when you give to them, they gather it up;
>   when you open your hand, they are filled with
>   good things.

When you hide your face, they are dismayed;
    when you take away their breath, they die
    and return to their dust.
When you send forth your spirit, they are created;
    and you renew the face of the ground
        (Ps 104:27-30).

The Natural World Is Good

"God saw everything that he had made, and indeed, it was very good" (Gen 1:31). Good, in Hebrew thinking, was not an ideal, but was seen in concrete experiences of God's actions. We experience God's goodness in the way he formed creation. Environmentalist Calvin DeWitt describes seven of the provisions God made for his creation: energy exchange, soil building, cycling (carbon cycle, hydrologic [water] cycle), water purification, creative fruitfulness, global circulation of water and air, and the human ability to learn from creation.[20]

Nurses experience nature's *goodness* all the time: when immune systems destroy invaders, when hearts pump effectively, when nervous systems conduct sensations and coordinate muscular movements, when eating good food causes children to grow and elders to work and play, when a loudly protesting infant is born healthy and with all her parts working. We rejoice in the goodness of nature when stress falls away in a mountain vacation. We depend on the goodness of nature to sustain us with water. Our very lives depend upon the goodness of the natural world.

It would be nice if we could stop at this point while thinking about the goodness of the natural world. But nurses also study pathophysiology. All is not well in the natural world, for in it we find sickness and death. Our environmental dwelling turns against us rather than supporting our lives. Those who advocate returning to nature because it is basically good are telling us some truth. The natural world is good because God created it that way. But they are not telling us the whole truth. Nature has no intentions toward us, benign or otherwise. When it sustains life it is working the way God meant it to. Even then, human involvement is required. For example, newborns left on their own die; nature does not care for them. Beyond that, we all know that even with the best of human care, nature doesn't always sustain life. Our work as nurses revolves around illness and death. Babies are born deformed. Accidents happen. Why does this contradiction in the natural world exist?

The Natural World Is in Bondage

So much of what happens seems *meaningless* and *unnatural*. A tornado suddenly rips through a community, leaving homes destroyed, hundreds of people admitted to emergency departments and dozens of people dead. A healthy young father falls into a grain bin as it is being filled; he smothers and dies. A home-health nurse loses the struggle to prevent amputating the limb of a middle-aged man with diabetes. A beautiful baby girl is stillborn because the umbilical cord was wrapped around her neck. A teenage boy dies years after receiving HIV-contaminated blood for treatment of hemophilia. A vibrant young teacher struggles daily with the invisible symptoms of fibromyalgia. Families live in temporary shelters awaiting the receding of flood waters that have destroyed their homes and farms. The stories go on and on.

The Bible tells us why things, including people, run down. It gives us some clues as to why there are sudden intrusions of death and suffering into our lives. Something is out of joint in the natural world. When the first humans rebelled against their dependence on God, the effects of that sin were devastating, not just for their relationship with God but for the natural world as well. God's original blessing of creation was reversed. He cursed the ground itself in judgment.[21]

Two effects of God's curse are the enslavement of nature and the entrance of death into the world. Animals, originally the joy and satisfaction of humans, now often became feared enemies. Work, which was to be creative and pleasurable, now became a struggle. Childbirth, meant to be joyous, became a painful experience. Human bodies, instead of supporting the eternal longings of our souls, will be torn from us in death, returning to the dust from which they are made (Gen 3:15-19).

Paradoxically, God's curse on the natural world was made in hope. Paul depicts creation as groaning in labor pains, pains that promise new life ahead. "Creation itself will be set free from its bondage to decay and will obtain the freedom of the glory of the children of God. We know that the whole creation has been groaning in labor pains until now" (Rom 8:21-22). In some way the liberation of nature from God's curse is tied up with human liberation in God's new creation.

Those who see nature as benign are blind to the frustration and decay of nature. They lay the problems of the natural world solely at the feet of human beings, blaming them for mismanagement and deliberate spoiling of the earth and its natural resources. Again, they are telling us some truth. Much that is wrong with our environment is due to human shortsightedness and greed.

Many blame Christianity for the present environmental crisis. Christianity teaches that God wants humanity—the pinnacle of his creative activity—to subdue the earth and have dominion over all living things (Gen 1:28). It is important to note that God told this to the first humans before they had rebelled against their Creator. When God told Adam and Eve to have dominion (Gen 1:28), the implication was that humans were to be God's agents and to care for creation.[22] We are to rule and subdue the natural world by serving it, not by exploiting it. Blaming Christianity itself for our present ecological crisis misses the problem. The problem is that humanity (including Christ's followers) has not been faithful and obedient to its calling.

Some thinkers today are realizing that humans themselves are fundamentally flawed, greedy and selfish. Rather than cooperatively caring for the natural environment, we hurry to take what we want and think little, if at all, of what others need. Eighteenth-century romantics like French philosopher Jean-Jacques Rousseau thought that human beings were intrinsically good until they were spoiled by civilization. Rousseau was an early advocate of the return to nature. Philosopher of science René Dubos counters such an optimistic view. He writes, "The fashionable view at present is that human nature was bad from the very beginning and civilization has only given wider ranges of expression to its fundamental bestiality."[23]

Nurses see people who suffer from environmental problems in every work setting: schools, clinics, community, physicians offices, emergency rooms, in-patient units. One classification of environmental health hazards includes living problems, work hazards, atmospheric quality, water quality, housing, food quality, waste control, radiation and violence.[24] Nurses working among the poor know that they bear a disproportionate risk of exposure to such hazards.

The Natural World Is to Be Cared For

In the midst of the frustrations and destruction of the natural world, God's word to us remains the same as it was to Adam and Eve, "Develop and care for creation." How can we obey this command in nursing? We begin by humbly recognizing our positions as God's agents in creation. There are at least two ways for nurses to do this: (1) by holding a humble, biblically informed view of technology and (2) by exercising our influence for care of the environment.

Those who decry technology are right in claiming that it often increases rather than relieves suffering. One of the reasons given for the increasing acceptance of physician-assisted suicide is the fear of being kept alive too long by machines. Aggressive use of technology often reflects a refusal to admit our inability to cure every condition and to always defeat death. The suffering person is lost from view in the race to solve the physiological puzzle.[25]

At the same time technology has given new ways to treat problems, enabled us to relieve pain, helped amputees walk. Who would want to give up using insulin? Even our stethoscopes are technology. Instead of rejecting technology as such, we need to struggle with the hard questions of when and how to use it.

Technology is an extension of human ability to develop and care for the natural world. Developing new technologies can be fulfilling God's calling. But there are dangers. One of the pitfalls to be avoided is transferring trust from God to technology. Ultimately God owns and sustains life. Pride denies our dependence on God and places it on human abilities. There are limits to what we can do, even with the most sophisticated technology. There are also limits to what we *should* do. It is always tempting to try everything possible to extend life—or to create new life. We need to learn when to stop.

We need to continually ask questions. Does our technology really benefit our patients? Is it motivated by a concern for the patient's good? Are we fair in the way we use technology? Is it available to all who need it or only to those who can afford it? Do a few people benefit from costly technology, leaving few resources for basic health care of the poor? Consider that most discussions about advanced technology occur in rich countries of the world. The questions of when and how to use ventilators rarely arise in poor nations, where the concerns are for the basics of clean water and enough food.

Struggling with such questions is never easy, and often there are no simple answers. But struggle we must. A recent conversation about high-tech medicine with a young radiologist skilled in the latest techniques of imaging is an example. He is a committed Christian seeking to bring his faith to bear on his work. He sometimes wonders if what he does contributes to the idea that this life is all there is. It's fine to try to keep people healthy, but how far should he go?

The story of Margaret and her husband, Roy, demonstrates trust in God's guiding and sustaining grace—combined with willingness to use good medical care. They had lived in a developing country as missionaries. During their stay Margaret contracted an amoebic liver infection. By all indications she recovered fully, and later she and her husband returned home with their two small sons.

Years later she developed cirrhosis of the liver, which could only be accounted for by the earlier amoebic infection. Over the years she had said that she did not want any extraordinary measures taken when she was dying, including transplants. Now came the test.

There was no hesitancy on her part. No, she would not consider transplantation. "I've had a good life, two fine sons, and I'm nearly seventy years old. I am not afraid to die. But then I might have ten years yet." However, she was willing to adjust her diet and to take medication to manage the ascites. She asked that the pastors and some of her close friends come to her home to anoint her with oil and pray for her. It was a moving time, full of love, tears and faith.

How long will Margaret live? No one knows for certain. But meanwhile she and her husband have built a smaller retirement home near their children and grandchildren. She does not talk much about her situation, so that people will not think of her as an invalid. She plans to live fully while she is living. Margaret's life is in God's hands.

We are not against transplants. The ability to give life to another through donating organs is a wonderful thing. Neither would Margaret and Roy rule out transplants as such. Roy is a physician and Margaret is a medical technologist. It is possible that they may even change their minds. But their story represents the kind of questioning we are suggesting.

Finally, we need to look and pray for creative ways to show concern for the natural environment. When we instruct patients how to dispose of needles and syringes properly, we are protecting the environment. When we press for changes in how institutions manage medical waste, we are preserving the environment. When we support community efforts to develop open spaces for parks and playgrounds, we are helping to sustain the vitality and beauty of the environment. When we participate in block clean-up programs we are serving creation. When we suggest reusable coffee cups instead of Styrofoam cups at work and in our churches, we are helping the landfill problem. When we press for fair-housing laws so that poor people can live in safe, pollution free homes, we are caring for the natural environment.

God, the Creator, alone is worthy of our loyalty and worship. He alone is the ultimate source of life and healing. Appropriately used, medications and technology can be God's gifts to us. But in the end they cannot give us life and ultimate satisfaction.

> God is our refuge and strength,
>   a very present help in trouble.
> Therefore we will not fear, though the earth should change,
>   though the mountains shake in the heart of
>   the sea. . . .
> "Be still and know that I am God!" (Ps 46:1-2, 10).

8

The Unseen
Environment

RUTH WORKED THE AFTERNOON SHIFT ON MAIN 3, A TELEM-
etry unit in a small community hospital. Many of the patients were elderly,
and most were seriously ill. She liked the challenge of making rapid and
accurate assessment of changes in their conditions and then responding to
help them. It was common for the same people to return again and again,
so she knew many of the patients and their families well. When patients
improved and returned home, she rejoiced. When they died she grieved, but
she enjoyed using the best of her nursing knowledge and skill. That was the
good part.

But there was another side. The head nurse of the unit was an insecure
and manipulative woman. She used her power to keep the staff on edge and
suspicious of one another. Besides that, most of Ruth's colleagues had
personal problems that kept them from concentrating on their work. A
nurse in the midst of sex-change procedures was dating the married unit
secretary. They later "married." One coworker had a husband in jail; others
were involved in affairs. There were several who had all the characteristics
of personality disorders. Gossip abounded—about each other, the administration, and patients. At one point Ruth estimated that of the thirty-five

people working on her unit, there were only five whose lives were relatively normal. The climate on the unit was stressful and confused. More than that, it was evil.

After several months, Ruth's supervisor asked her to be the regular evening charge nurse. She accepted because she thought God had placed her in this situation for a reason. She saw her responsibility as mentoring the team leaders, some of whom had little idea of how to manage the nursing assistants and LPNs working on their teams. Soon everyone knew that Ruth had no time for prolonged gossiping in the utility room. Further, they knew that she would hold them accountable for their assignments. She was tough, but she was also fair. The word got back to Ruth that everyone liked working when she was in charge. There was still the problem with the head nurse. But eventually she was asked to resign. The nurse dating the unit secretary was transferred to another unit. Life on Main 3 was far from perfect, but it was a lot better than when Ruth began.

What was going on in the environment on Main 3? In the modernist worldview, the problem would be defined as lack of proper orientation of staff and inadequate leadership by the head nurse. A nurse working from New Paradigm thinking might say that energy was unbalanced. Perhaps someone who knew *feng shui* would suggest rearranging the furniture in the nurses' station or painting the walls another color. Correcting these problems could be useful; maybe even rearranging the work stations would help. But the underlying problem was evil, evil in the relationships of the staff. In the biblical view the environment on Main 3 went beyond psychological or social explanations. Ruth's leadership helped to eliminate unrighteous patterns and bring about order and productive working relationships. She brought God's *shalom* to Main 3.

My own (Arlene's) experience in home health care brought me face to face with the unseen in a different way. I went into homes where family life was so discordant that children were spoken to only in harsh language if they were addressed at all, where no one read stories to children, and where children bearing children were so overwhelmed that they spent their days watching TV. Attempts to teach a better way seemed almost futile. Where should one begin? After watching well-intentioned government programs pour money into community-based programs for many years with little noticeable improvement in the lives of people, one comes to realize that the problems are much too large to be fixed by programs.[1]

Another story represents the positive side of the unseen environment. Over a period of several years I went with students in home health to see an elderly woman being cared for by her daughter. A stroke had taken away the mother's ability to speak. She spent her days in bed completely helpless. The faithful care of her daughter was given at great cost of time and effort, but she would have not considered another way. I never asked her why she did it. I knew. Her Christian faith taught her responsibility for her parent and gave her strength to endure year after year. On some visits we talked of the Lord's sustaining grace.

Things in the unseen environment are seen by faith. They are realities not perceived by the five senses that serve us well in our space-time environment. Nurses have always known when observing birth, suffering and death that there is something about people that goes beyond the physical body—something not explainable by physics. We see evidence of this in the courage and faith of the mother with multiple sclerosis whose husband has left her, out of frustration with her handicaps. We see it in the mother of a boy killed in a gang fight when she forgives those who shot him.

In chapter seven we considered the natural environment, the seen world that can be weighed and measured. In this chapter we turn to the unseen environment, the world that can be perceived only indirectly. According to the modern worldview, we can know only the seen natural world, and human behavior can best be explained by the physical and social sciences. Many of those who adopt the postmodern position would agree with Christians that an unseen world exists. Recently a convention of Ghost Hunters was held not far from my (Arlene's) home. Members use instruments that detect electromagnetic fields, cameras with special film and other instruments to confirm their belief that ghosts inhabit certain locations. Historical buildings and sites are most likely to be haunted, they say. The Bible, however, gives us no reason to go looking for ghosts (spirits of departed persons). In fact, it strictly forbids us to do so (Deut 18:10-11).

If the unseen world is only indirectly perceived from the seen world, how can we learn about it? How do we interpret events that seem to relate to it? Is there a way to know truth about the unseen environment? Is one person's idea as good as another? Some would say so. To answer these questions we turn to Scripture.

God's Revelation of the Unseen Environment

The unseen environment is the spiritual aspect of creation. The unseen is where God dwells (Jn 1:18). It is also inhabited by personal beings, embodied and disembodied, human and nonhuman. It is the moral place where we find God's law, the foundation of morality. The unseen realm is where we find things that are eternal. Paul wrote, "What can be seen is temporary, but what cannot be seen is eternal" (2 Cor 4:18). We have a deep longing for the eternal even though our natural lives will end in death (Eccles 3:11).[2] These unseen realities are the most important aspects of our lives. Life without them is "vanity and chasing after wind" (Eccles 4:16). But if we cannot see them, how can we know about them?

According to the modern worldview there is no way to have certain knowledge of these things; we can only speculate about what they might be, if they exist at all. Since that is the case, we need to get on with practical realities that can be seen and known through science. We are given facts with no meaning, technical and political power with no morality, and human life with only practical value.

Those who fit into a more postmodern way of thinking tell us that each person must find her or his own spiritual truth. The way to do this is through intuition or various mystical experiences. Examples include accounts of near-death experiences in which we are given descriptions of supernatural beings and their messages. This approach, however, leaves us totally unconnected to actual events in the seen world. We are left to each person's own imagination and experience, an unreliable way to learn the truth.

The search for spiritual understanding is ancient. Job asked, "Where then does wisdom come from? And where is the place of understanding?" (Job 28:20). Ezekiel condemned those who gave prophecies out of their own imagination (Ezek 13:2). Human minds can produce futile thinking, and wisdom can be turned to foolishness (Rom 1:21-22). Moral thinking becomes debased, leading to all manner of evil and debauchery (Rom 1:28-31). Paul warned sophisticated Greek pagans, "We ought not to think that the deity is like gold, or silver, or stone, an image formed by the art and imagination of mortals" (Acts 17:29). John counsels us to not believe every spiritual message (1 Jn 4:1). With Job we ask, "Where can wisdom be found?"

Wisdom dwells with God. Isaiah the prophet wrote, "Have you not known? Have you not heard? The LORD is the everlasting God, the Creator of the ends of the earth. He does not faint or grow weary; his understanding is unsearchable" (Is 40:28). The way to spiritual understanding begins with reverence and love for God and willingness to walk in his ways. "The fear of the LORD is the beginning of wisdom, and the knowledge of the Holy One is insight" (Prov 9:10).

Because God is personal and we too are personal, it is possible for God to communicate with us. When creation was new, God walked and talked with humans in an open and direct way. They walked together in the cool of the evening. But the disobedience of the man and woman broke that open relationship (Gen 3:1-24). Since then God's communication with humans has come in different, more hidden ways. But he continues to speak.

How does God speak? He reveals his heart and mind to us in ways similar to the way we tell each other about ourselves. The Bible tells us that God sometimes speaks directly to people in dreams and visions (Joel 2:28). God also reveals himself through his actions. When we become aware of the divine significance of actual events, we learn something of God. David and Karen Mains call watching for God in our daily lives "the God hunt" and seeing evidence of him "God sightings."[3]

Jesus Christ, however, is God's most complete revelation of himself. "No one has ever seen God. It is God the only Son, who is close to the Father's heart, who has made him known" (Jn 1:18). "All other revelations and illuminations are simply clarifications and/or affirmations of this one incomparable revelation in human history."[4] Jesus told one of his disciples who asked to see the Father, "Have I been with you all this time, Philip, and you still do not know me? Whoever has seen me has seen the Father. How can you say, 'Show us the Father'?" (Jn 14:9).

The Bible is the inspired witness of those who heard and experienced God's various revelations of himself. Its central theme is Jesus Christ. The Bible is the primary means God uses to break through our darkness and sin to bring us hope and light. It gives us a perspective for seeing the unseen in the everyday happenings of our lives. It helps us to know that things are not what they appear to be, viewed from the seen world only. It gives us criteria for "testing the spirits," for judging the validity of various spiritual experiences that people have.[5]

The church hands down the interpretation of Scripture from one generation to another. However, "none of us can actually know the word of God until God personally reveals himself to us. When God speaks we will know it, for his word is 'living and active, sharper than any two-edged sword'" (Heb 4:12).[6]

"The Bible is a prism by which the light of God shines on us."[7] God's Spirit interprets the words of Scripture to us and awakens us to the significance of Jesus Christ for our lives. It is Jesus Christ who reveals God to us.

God's self-communication to us is called *revelation*. Theologian Donald Bloesch describes revelation this way:

> Revelation is indeed cognitive, but it is much more than this. It is an act of communication by which God confronts the whole person with his redeeming mercy and glorious presence. It therefore involves not only the mind but also the will and affections.[8]

When God speaks, he does not permit us a neutral position. We must choose to either accept his word and do what he tells us or reject his word and rebel against him. It is an awesome thing to hear God speak. But when we receive his word with a humble and obedient heart, God teaches us wisdom. "He leads the humble in what is right, and teaches the humble his way" (Ps 25:9).

When we receive God's revelation in faith, he opens our inner (spiritual) eyes to a transcendent dimension of reality, the unseen environment. The Scriptures refer often to eyes and ears of the heart. Paul prayed for spiritual vision for believers in Ephesus:

I pray that the God of our Lord Jesus Christ, the Father of glory, may give you a spirit of wisdom and revelation as you come to know him, so that, with the eyes of your heart enlightened, you may know what is the hope to which he has called you, what are the riches of his glorious inheritance among the saints, and what is the immeasurable greatness of his power for us who believe, according to the working of his great power. (Eph 1:17-19)

Paul was not interested in spiritual vision just out of curiosity or as a way to gain spiritual power. God mercifully shields us from much in the unseen world, showing us only those things necessary for our salvation. "The secret things belong to the LORD our God, but the revealed things belong to us and to our children forever, to observe all the words of this law" (Deut 29:29). God opens our spiritual eyes so that we can know him, his love and holiness. We also need to have our spiritual eyes opened to understand who we really are: created in God's image yet corrupted at the deepest level by sin. Spiritual vision helps to see our need for redemption and salvation, not just enlightenment, education and social reform.

Knowing God's will must be expressed in godly moral living. Paul prayed for the Christians at Colossae "that you may be filled with the knowledge of God's will in all spiritual wisdom and understanding, so that you may lead lives worthy of the Lord, fully pleasing to him, as you bear fruit in every good work and as you grow in the knowledge of God" (Col 1:9-10). Spiritual vision is given to help us understand more of God in order to please and honor him. As God's Spirit gives us both understanding and spiritual strength, our very character will be changed. We exhibit the fruit of the Spirit (Gal 5:22-23) and experience *shalom* personally and in our lives together (Is 32:17).

It is possible, however, to resist God's revelation, to close our eyes and ears, to harden our hearts. Paul quoted the prophet Isaiah when referring to those who refused to accept the message of Jesus that Paul preached.

Go to this people and say,
You will indeed listen, but never understand,
    and you will indeed look, but never perceive.

For this people's heart has grown dull,
  and their ears are hard of hearing,
    and they have shut their eyes;
    so that they might not look with their eyes,
  and listen with their ears,
and understand with their heart and turn—
  and I would heal them. (Acts 28:26-27)

To be without spiritual vision and hearing is spiritual death. Paul contrasted the lives of people who followed the Holy Spirit with those who followed what he called the *flesh*: "fornication, impurity, licentiousness, idolatry, sorcery, enmities, strife, jealousy, anger, quarrels, dissensions, factions, envy, drunkenness, carousing, and things like these. I am warning you, as I warned you before: those who do such things will not inherit the kingdom of God" (Gal 5:19-21). "Flesh" here does not mean our physical bodies but rather living only by what can be seen in the natural world and closing our hearts to God.

The experience of Ruth and her coworkers on Main 3 is an example of how the works of the flesh bring chaos to a nursing unit. It also shows us how the fruit of the Spirit in Ruth's life affected the climate of the whole unit. Main 3 reflected the ongoing, unseen spiritual struggle.

The Struggle in the Unseen Environment

What is going on in this unseen world? The Scriptures tell us of a struggle between two kingdoms. Each of them, the kingdom of this world and the kingdom of God, are competing for citizens. The outcome of this struggle is secure: the heavenly kingdom will prevail.[9] The decisive battle has been fought and won by the death and resurrection of Jesus Christ. But God, for his own reasons, has permitted follow-up battles to continue. The ruler of the "worldly kingdom,"[10] Satan, was once a powerful angel in God's presence. The Scriptures allude to a heavenly rebellion in which Satan lost his privileged position after trying to assume God's powers. Still powerful, he now rules over a large number of evil beings who plot with him against God's kingdom and its citizens.[11]

His power, however, is deception, not truth. "The devil and his hosts are not gods, but they pretend to be so. They are really "feeble and bankrupt elemental spirits (Gal 4:9) and their power is that of the lie" (Jn 8:44).[12] One of their primary tactics is working to deceive us about the truth of God (2 Cor 4:3-4).

The first story of human rebellion in the Garden of Eden recounts just such an act of treacherous deceit in which the serpent put doubts about God's love and goodness into the minds of Adam and Eve. He suggested that they should make their own decisions about good and evil rather than trust the Creator (Gen 3:1-5). He challenged them to reach for powers that were reserved for God alone. This is the core of the struggle that continues to this day in the unseen world. People, mere creatures, are trying to live as if they were not dependent upon a loving Creator. Human autonomy may seem good at first, but it is a deception from the enemy, and eventually everything goes wrong. In truth, unless we give our loyalty to God and his kingdom we remain as prisoners in what Scripture calls "the power of darkness" (Col 1:13).[13] The Bible calls rebellion against God sin.

The effects of sin and rebellion are everywhere around us—violence, confusion in sexuality, alienation in families and communities, oppressive social structures. A great number of the social causes of disease identified by the NIH Committee referred to in chapter seven are spiritually rooted. How much can nursing, or even the whole health care system, do about family violence and sexual abuse? Nursing deals with the symptoms and has some success. But the root problems lie elsewhere, somewhere outside the world that can be controlled by science.

Effects of the Unseen in Society

In the Genesis story of humanity's first rebellion against their loving Creator, we find the seeds of all the destruction caused by sin: fear of God rather than trust; shame with nakedness, alienation between men and women; fear between humans and animals, pain in childbearing; frustration in work, death (Gen 3:8-24). Soon we learn of the first murder, when Cain killed his brother, Abel, and later we read of the continued effects of human revenge (Gen 4). This is the human story, and it occurs over and over again throughout history.

James Boice identifies the social effects of trying to build human society apart from dependence upon the loving Creator God: (1) a loss of roots and a restlessness; (2) closeness without community; (3) idolatrous worship of physical beauty; (4) pride in power and violent strength.[14] Boice refers to Simone Weil's conclusion that "the only cure for uprootedness is a rediscovery of the human being as God's creature and of God himself as the source of those basic elements without which a proper civilization cannot function: order, liberty, obedience, responsibility, equality, the right to express one's opinion, security, private property, truth and others." "She was exactly right," says Boice. "Our only true roots are in God."[15] Like that of our biblical ancestors, our culture today is increasingly hard, arrogant, self-seeking and violent.

Nurses recognize the results of living independently from God in their work. The busyness and restless activity characterizing our lives are often attempts to camouflage the terror of rootlessness. How many of the stress-related diseases that nurses both experience and treat have their roots in such restlessness? Stress-management practices that fail to deal with the root problem are like feeble attempts to staunch massive bleeding with Band-Aids.

People live in close proximity in today's urban culture. Yet they are lonely. We see the symptoms of loneliness in people who turn to drugs and alcohol for escape. Others call hot lines late at night to hear the voice of someone telling them why they should not commit suicide.

Our culture idolizes those having perfect bodies and sexual charm. Even though some women protest against it, beauty is marketed in pageants and goods are sold by sexually explicit advertising. "But [women] will continue to be exploited in the worst way and will even willingly submit to that exploitation until they discover that they are creatures made in the image of God, not of the latest rock star or movie idol."[16] The thousands of young people struggling with anorexia and bulimia are slaves to this lie.

Finally, our culture is increasingly marked by worship of raw power, with a resulting increase in violence and crime. Nurses working in emergency departments, both rural and urban, can attest to this. We see the struggle for power in the politics of health care, both at the unit and agency level and in the larger arena of professional and economic maneuvering for control. Author Cheryl Forbes writes that the point of power is to be visible.[17] How much energy is spent today on image-building and "power dressing"? It is present even in nursing. We are certainly not opposed to looking smart and dressing well. But when service and substance get lost in the drive for power, then power is wielding us.

We do not like to think of life in this way. Modern people have long thought that human progress on all fronts was inevitable, that we merely had to cooperate with the inevitable by gaining more knowledge and providing better education. Even today, when the myth of progress has been exposed as a lie and many despair of the future of humanity, we still do not like to think about sin.[18] We label human behavior sick rather than evil, except when the evidence is so overwhelming that it cannot be ignored, such as the massacre of thousands for "ethnic cleansing."[19] Then the problem is usually in "those people," often in other countries. We do not like to think of ourselves as sinful, as persons capable of morally twisted behavior and selfishness.[20] But morally twisted behavior is the end result of living apart from God and thus as slaves to sin (Rom 8:15-17).

Moral Certainties in the Unseen Environment

To this point we have considered the way the unseen is expressed in social behavior. Our relationships and interactions have moral implications. Understanding another aspect of the unseen, the moral dimension, is critical. Nursing today is searching for a moral anchor, but like the culture around us there is no acceptable agreement as to what that is. Legal, social, traditional and professional criteria are variously put forth as the place to begin. Some nurse ethicists, wanting a more enduring foundation, argue for natural law ethics. Others are turning to an ethic of care. All these ethics begin in the seen world and are based on human experience or reason. Nursing, now considered a secular profession, cannot accept a religious foundation for its ethics. Would recovery of our spiritual vision help us? We believe that it would.

Philosophers and unsophisticated people in all ages and places recognize a moral reality (Rom 1:19-23).

Because we live in a moral universe created by God, it is not strange that wise people throughout history have discovered universal-moral principles like justice, benevolence and truth. How often have you cried out in the midst of a frustrating situation, "That's not fair!" There wasn't time for deep theological reflection. The feeling just came from your gut. Aristotle observed that we know what justice is when we feel the wounds of injustice.[21]

The moral aspect of creation is not only "out there"; it is within us as well. God created us in his likeness, and our moral calling is to express God's character. "The law of God for our behavior corresponds with the way we are made and with the world in which he asks us to be moral agents."[22] Those who advocate a *natural law* ethic are right when they argue for a moral creation. Paul writes about those who do instinctively what God's law requires because it is written on their hearts (Rom 2:14-15).

Reflecting on our general sense of morality, however, leaves us perplexed. What does natural law tell us? What does it mean to be kind and just? Those who advocate assisted suicide, for example, sprinkle their arguments with the word *compassion*. Justice means different things to people. Furthermore, we do not do even the good we know to do; our wills are bound (Rom 1:15-16). We are then not only perplexed, we are guilt-ridden as well. We need more than a moral creation. We need a moral Creator.

Christians believe that morality is rooted in the character of God. God is a God of justice and righteousness, love and mercy. "Righteousness and justice are the foundation of your throne; steadfast love and faithfulness go before you" (Ps 89:14). God's law meets our need for moral understanding. "The law of the LORD is perfect, reviving the soul; the decrees of the LORD are sure, making wise the simple" (Ps 19:7). God's law does not change (Ps 33:11; 119:152). God's law is true. "The sum of your word is truth; and every one of your righteous ordinances endures forever" (Ps 119:160). God's word teaches us the distinction between good and evil (Heb 5:14; Rom 12:2). Finally, God's law observed brings a life of *shalom*. "Great peace have those who love your law; nothing can make them stumble" (Ps 119:165).

Ethicist John Kilner describes a biblical ethic for health care that brings together the best of other ethical theories. He identifies his approach as *God-centered, reality-bounded* and *love-impelled.*

A God-centered ethic begins with who God is, what his purposes for us are and what his image in people looks like. Because our reasoning is both limited and sinful, we need more than ethical principles—we need a Guide, the Holy Spirit, to help us discern the complex issues we face, and we need moral strength to do what is right.

The reality boundaries define good and evil for us and give us moral guidance for the various aspects of our lives. Here Kilner includes such things as contributing to the needs of others and viewing people as holy ones to be treated with special care. Kilner identifies four ethical guides as especially pertinent for health care: (1) promoting life, (2) acting justly, (3) freedom and (4) telling the truth. There are times when we are not sure what should be done in specific situations. Then we need to discern how to apply these guides. Our Guide, the Holy Spirit, helps us.

Finally, a biblical ethic is love-impelled, building others up and helping them to experience as much good as possible. Neighbor love is expressed in community and takes into account how our actions will affect others.[23]

Nurses struggling with the moral implications of a health care system driven by economic profit are reflecting God's moral concern for justice. When we cry out against injustice in the care of the poor we are expressing God's moral indignation. When coping with ethical issues relating to arrogant use of technology, we need to remember that we are accountable to God. Patients and caregivers wanting total control over the beginning and end of life are grasping for an autonomy that God did not give to us. In the morally uncertain climate today, nursing needs to recover its spiritual vision. We need a God-centered ethic.

Nurses and the Unseen Environment

The unseen environment has vast implications for nursing. In the above discussion we have touched on the social and moral implications. Now we conclude by identifying several practical ways that we can live wisely in this environment as nurses.

First of all, we can actively seek biblical wisdom. One author has coined the phrase *godliness in working clothes.*[24] Scripture gives us much practical wisdom for relating to patients and coworkers, for conducting ourselves with those in authority and for doing our work in an ethical way.

Second, we need to remember that we are in a spiritual battle with evil. When relationships in our work are devious and confused, we need to be aware that we are not fighting against certain people so much as against unseen spiritual beings. We are given spiritual weapons for this battle: truth, righteousness, peace, faith, salvation, Scripture and prayer (Eph 6:10-18).

We also have good news to bring to our patients and coworkers, news that we can learn only from God's revelation of himself in Jesus Christ. It is good news that pushes back the kingdom of darkness and fear that holds many of our patients and coworkers in its grip. In a later chapter we will consider how to give spiritual care—how to share this good news.

Another practical consideration concerns the truth that things are not always what they seem. Knowing this has significance for nursing research. Nursing is moving more and more to qualitative research methods to capture the personal nature of caring. The frameworks through which we perceive and interpret nursing phenomena are derived from particular understandings of the unseen. Christian nurses will want to make such frameworks explicit and then evaluate them based on biblical and theological knowledge. For example, most nursing research assumes an understanding about the person. We want to ask, How does this view compare to what the Bible teaches us about people? This is not to say that we cannot learn some truth from theories not explicitly Christian, but it does mean that we need to be clear about the limitations of the interpretive frameworks we use. We need to discard those that give us a totally wrong understanding.

Keeping Our Focus

Finally a word of hope. Our environment abounds with evidence of sin and evil. But there is good news. As socially devastating as sin is, it is not the most important side of the struggle in the unseen environment. The universe is still God's creation. We pointed out at the beginning of this section that the decisive battle in the unseen struggle has already been won by Jesus Christ. The evidence is an empty cross and an empty tomb on the first

Easter. God is still present and acting. Eugene Peterson writes:

> We live on holy ground. We inhabit sacred space. This holy ground is subject to incredible violations. This sacred space suffers constant sacrilege. No matter—the holiness is there, the sacredness is there. If our lives, and in this case our caring, are shaped in response to the violations, to the sacrilege, and not out of the holy, they are shaped wrongly.[25]

In this light Peterson counsels us to be restrained in our acts of caring because caring—"responding to a person in need—takes place in an environment already surging with life, prodigal with energy, vitality, beauty."[26] He calls us to worship, to stop our activity of caring long enough to discover what God is doing. Those of us who care for others should look for God in every situation.

Each day we need to ask God to open our eyes to see him acting, our ears to hear him speaking to us—through our patients, through those with whom we work, through the often confused or evil situations in which we find ourselves. We do this by taking time to let God first speak to us in his Word so that our vision is clearer and our hearing more acute. We do this through private and corporate worship. We do it through hearing the counsel of other nurses who also walk with God. These are all ways to heed Paul's words to keep our focus on what God is doing in our environment (Col 3:2). We can then enter each day knowing that we are not alone, for God is with us.

9

A Storied Environment

ELAINE STRUGGLED WITH AN INNER PROMPTING THAT SHE thought was God's voice: *Go talk to the patient in room 321.* She was not at all eager to enter the room. The patient, Mary Ann, had been admitted to the surgical unit after a suicide attempt. Elaine had little experience with such patients and was fearful of saying or doing the wrong thing. Finally she had a short break in her work and went to 321. Elaine felt that God gave her a special boldness as she asked Mary Ann why she had tried to take her life. "My husband said he doesn't love me anymore, and he wants a divorce," Mary Ann said dejectedly.

At that moment Elaine knew why God had urged her to go into this room. "Five months before, my husband had said the same words to me. I knew the pain of hearing those words, and I could identify with her desperation." When it seemed clear that Mary Ann did not want to say more, Elaine shared her own story, all the while feeling odd telling a stranger her problem. But she could tell that Mary Ann seemed eager to hear more. "Did you get a divorce?" she asked.

"No, we didn't," Elaine said. "He decided that he was confused when he said it, and he wants to try again. I have prayed that God will help me forgive him, and we are depending on God to heal our marriage." She then identified herself as a Christian believer.

"I'm a Christian too," said Mary Ann. "But my husband moved out."

Elaine wished that she could assure Mary Ann that her husband would come back, that everything would be fine, that God would heal their marriage and they would live happily ever after. "All I could do was remind her what a powerful God we have, and that although her husband had left her, God hadn't."

Then she had to leave because her patient from surgery had returned to the unit. "I'll be praying for you," she said to Mary Ann and gently squeezed her hand.

Elaine wrote this story for the *Journal of Christian Nursing* seventeen years later, after celebrating her nineteenth wedding anniversary. She concluded with the following paragraph:

> I didn't know much about caring for suicidal patients, but I discovered that day that God does. Sometimes in nursing, he calls us to listen to his voice and obey, because he knows everything about our patients. He knows their deep needs better than we do. He knew that Mary Ann needed to know that she was not alone, that even other Christians were suffering the same pain she was. She needed someone to remind her that God will bring us through every crisis life has to offer. I felt grateful and privileged that he used me to pass on his hope to her.[1]

The hope Elaine offered to Mary Ann was not a bland optimism that things always work out. Her own pain prevented her from doing that. The hope she offered was in the God of hope, the God who works to achieve his purposes in our lives, often in ways unseen.

Nurses have always been bearers of hope by their words and by their acts of caring. As we saw earlier, nursing was taken around the world by Christian missionaries who often worked with few resources. Nurse historian Linda Sabin cites the example of Mrs. Charles Lewis, a missionary nurse in China. Mrs. Lewis put the following notice in a 1915 *American Journal of Nursing:*

We are looking for two or three more good, conscientious nurses who are anxious to be useful in laying the foundations for reliable nursing in the future China. Thirty-two hundred patients were seen at our clinics in Pautingfu last year, and 823 operations were done, and yet, we must beg for nurses to go and help with this work.[2]

Christian missionaries obey the words Christ spoke before ascending to heaven: "Go therefore and make disciples of all nations, baptizing them in the name of the Father, and of the Son and of the Holy Spirit, and teaching them to obey everything that I have commanded you. And remember, I am with you always, to the end of the age" (Mt 28:19-29). Along with their preaching, missionaries have offered practical actions to make life better for those they were serving.[3] Christ's command and the promise of his presence have enabled them to continue their work as bearers of hope.

Defining Hope

Mary Thompson, whose research focused on nurturing hope in patients, defines hope in this way:

Hope is the expectation of attaining a goal, the knowledge and feeling that there is a way out of difficulty. It is a perspective on life that results in action. Hope enables a person facing a potentially despairing situation not to give up.[4]

Hope expects new things to happen in the future. Life isn't just the same old thing over and over. Growth and progress are possible.

Hope has always been a vital aspect of nursing, for both nurses and their patients. The hopeful nurse finds strength to continue working in the face of great odds. Common nursing wisdom tells us that patients who have hope improve physically and emotionally more often than those without hope. Nurses were among the first to do research on how hope affects the healing process.[5] We have hope that, even though it may take some time, treatments will be effective. We urge our patients to hope that medications will work, that surgery will be beneficial, that exercise will improve muscle strength. We encourage them to trust the skill of their caregivers. We help them find hope, in the face of crippling disease, for some improvement or for slowing their decline. Just being alive is reason for hope. Death is the end of hope, at least for this life.

Whistling in the Dark?

Nurses write much about the benefits of hope. But what if we can no longer offer hope that improvement is possible or that our nursing interventions will help? For example, how could Elaine offer hope to Mary Ann concerning her marriage when there seemed to be no hope for it? Often it seems we are urged to "hope in hope." The positive psychological benefits of hope are stressed. But why should anyone hope for a better future when all evidence belies the possibility? Are we merely "whistling in the dark"?

Two theorists who have influenced nursing, one a nurse and the other a developmental psychologist, are examples of unfounded optimism. Martha Rogers was one of the first to explicitly include the time dimension in nursing theory. Time, the fourth dimension, adds a sense of movement and liveliness to her nursing theory.[6] By including this fourth dimension of time, Rogers opened new ways of thinking about nursing. In her view increasing complexity, diversity and rhythmicity of the life process were inevitable and good.[7] Her ideas appealed to many when she first proposed them, and they still do. Rogers's theory is optimistic. It assumes that people and societies always move over time in a positive direction.[8]

Erik Erikson's *Childhood and Society*, published in 1950, was the impetus for nursing's interest in the life-cycle, first taken up in psychiatric and pediatric texts and eventually spreading throughout the entire curriculum. Erikson proposed his theory at a time when psychology and sociology were eagerly accepted as means to create a new humanity capable of living in harmony rather then always being at war. Erikson's optimistic interpretation of Darwinian theory shapes his psychosocial theory.

Both Martha Rogers and Erik Erikson were basically hopeful about the future. Erikson, born in 1902 in Europe, and Rogers, born in 1914 in the American South, lived in the years when the "myth of progress" was beginning to weaken in intellectual circles. Yet the dying of a cultural assumption is prolonged, and both of them, along with many others in academia, continued to express this optimism. Historian Roy Swanstrom characterizes the "cult of progress" this way:

> The experts were not thoroughly agreed about what progress meant, but the general feeling was that year by year, century by century, mankind was moving toward the day when material well-being would replace poverty and deprivation; rationality would replace myth and superstition; liberty and democracy would replace despotism and tyranny; a world-wide human brotherhood would replace hatred and war; and humanity would be the ruler rather than the victim of the forces of nature. Note the implication that while the conditions of life are constantly improving in quality, the human race itself is growing in both virtue and wisdom.[9]

Lillian Wald is an example from nursing history of one who practiced this belief in human progress. Along with Mary Brewster, she founded the Henry Street Settlement House in 1893 on New York City's Lower East Side. She was a strong believer that public health nursing would assist human progress by applying scientific knowledge. Forty years after founding Henry Street she could write the following:

> Increasing emphasis is laid on detecting and overcoming defects in children—cardiac, dental, visual, aural, and others. In this effort it may be repeated that the nurse is the indispensable interpreter of the aims and methods of modern medical science.[10]

Wald was an enthusiastic supporter of the newly developing field of "mental hygiene" and taught the Henry Street nurses to secure treatment for mentally ill members of the families in their care. She also believed that "in the nurse's approach to her cases, she needs to know the fundamentals of modern psychology so that her own relationship with them may be sound and productive."[11] Wald's passion was progress in human relations in the broadest sense, and she saw education, supported by government policy, as the means for social engineering. She did not expect miracles but "something better—the opportunity to work out for ourselves a planned and controlled way of life."[12] The ideals of public health nursing today still reflect Wald's century-old vision.[13]

Others shared this hope for the benefits of public health. A 1949 textbook of hygiene and public health even promotes "the control of racial health through the application of a knowledge of heredity and through sex hygiene."[14] Such an optimistic view of eugenics in 1949 is frightening. Where was the writer when the work of Nazi physicians in concentration camps were revealed to the world in 1945? Was he naive, or did he approve?

The Decline of the Myth of Progress

Why was the idea of progress so prevalent? Scholars attribute this attitude to the Enlightenment and the secularization of a biblical understanding of human history. According to theologian Robert Jenson, Westerners have understood human life as realistic narrative. We think that the sequence of events in our life should make a certain kind of "dramatic sense" because they fit within a real *universal* story.

Today many have lost faith in the idea that our lives should make sense within a larger story. The reason is that "modernity was defined by the attempt to live in a universal story without a universal storyteller." Jenson explains:

> The entire project of the Enlightenment was to maintain realist faith while declaring disallegiance from the God who was that faith's object. The story the Bible tells is asserted to be the story of God with His creatures; that is, it is both assumed and explicitly asserted that there is a true story about the universe because there is a universal novelist/historian.[15]

We see the effects of "disallegiance from God" in society. God, no longer taken seriously in public life, is relegated to private life. We explain the natural world and human life without reference to God. Modern science has *desacralized* the environment—pushed gods and demons out of the human dwelling. By contrast, in many cultures, past and present, the environment itself is considered *sacred*. Everything has religious significance and "every human experience is capable of being transfigured, lived on a different, a transhuman plane."[16] In the modern worldview people must create significance for their own lives.

But living without God as the "universal storyteller" is a project doomed to fail. Two world wars, continuing revolutions and military actions, and "cleansings" of various sorts—ethnic, social and political—have shattered utopian dreams of progress. Rising crime rates, government scandals, family breakdown and the widening gap between rich and poor undermine optimism for the future. Our accumulation of material comforts and our technological advances have not been accompanied by the expected moral improvement. As a result, many today see human history as meaningless, without story. "If there is no God, or indeed if there is some other God than the God of the Bible, there is no narratable world," writes Jenson.[17]

This loss of a sense of meaningful history affects not only humanity as a whole. Many today have lost hope that their personal lives have any significance. For a time we can live *as if* things will indeed work out for the better. But then reality hits. Erikson's theory provides a stark example. His work locates personal identity within human culture and society. But he gives us no larger story and no universal story teller. After the final stage of development comes death and the end of one's identity.[18]

Nurses see this loss of story in patients who are self-destructive, who live with no hope and no goals, who are indeed afraid to hope. They see it in patients whose personal identity is confused. They see it in fellow nurses whose frantic attempts to find meaning in life are self-demeaning and destructive: multiple sexual affairs, partying, debt-accumulating shopping sprees. They see it in patients (and themselves) suffering from stress-related health problems because they are "seeking immortality through work."[19] They see it in the growing demand for legal access to assisted suicide when loss and illness threaten patients' identity as competent and capable individuals in control of their lives. Living without a story is a terrifying thing.

Returning to God's Story

Would returning to the biblical story help nursing to find a source of hope? We believe so! Is such a return a regression to the past? We believe it is a return to reality! The Bible tells a grand and true story, God's story of redeeming his creation and rescuing humanity from captivity to sin and its effects. Rather than evolutionary human progress, the Bible tells us of a perfect creation from which humanity fell. But God is rewriting the story of human rebellion and sin with a new conclusion. He is creating a new humanity, a new kingdom.

The biblical idea that human history is linear—has a beginning and an end, purpose and direction—contrasts starkly with other views both ancient and modern: (1) chaotic views in which the human story has no purpose, pattern or significance; (2) circular or cyclical views in which life is merely an endless repetition of cycles, sometimes called the eternal return; (3) mechanical views in which humans are merely products of nature with no freedom or possibility of change; (4) progressive or developmental views in which human institutions and thought emerge naturally from the simple to the complex over the course of time. In the biblical worldview, human history has a course and moves toward a goal *not inherent* in the nature of things. The goal is outside history, in God's own purposes. God's superintending of human history as well as sustaining the natural world is called *providence:* "God's faithful and effective care and guidance of everything which He has made toward the end which He has chosen."[20]

What are God's plans and purposes for humanity? First we must understand that they are beyond our ability to discover through reason or experience alone. God is unlimited and holy in his understanding and ways. We are limited and sinful. Our minds are simply incapable of fully comprehending God's mind and of interpreting our lives. If we are to know God's purposes, God must reveal them to us (Is 55:8-9). In fact, he wants us to ask him about his ways, so that he may help us understand his grand story.[21]

In chapters seven and eight we said that there is trouble in God's creation. God's story is not one of bland optimism in which evil is ignored or discounted. But—in contrast to the best of human plans—God's unchanging plans and purposes will be fulfilled in spite of his rebellious creatures.[22]

> For I am God, and there is no other;
>   I am God, and there is no one like me,
> declaring the end from the beginning
>   and from ancient times things not yet done,

saying, "My purpose shall stand,
   and I will fulfill my intention. . . .
I have spoken, and I will bring it to pass;
   I have planned, and I will do it. (Is 46:9-11)

What is the story God tells us? In the Bible we read of God's creating a new humanity, those who live under his reign. He is creating a new kingdom in which his laws are not imposed from the outside but come from the hearts of its citizens (Ezek 36:27). Further, God himself will live among his people (Rev 21:3), and God himself will banish hostility and violence. No abusive spouses will rip families apart. No rabid dogs will bite children, and no deadly viruses will sap life (Is 11:6-9).

Jesus of Nazareth is the central figure in God's new story. With the birth of Jesus in Bethlehem two thousand years ago, God opened the possibility of a new relationship between God and people. Jesus, conceived by the Holy Spirit, carried in the womb of Mary, born in an animal stable, was the long awaited Messiah, God's anointed one, coming to save his creation. God entered human history, becoming fully human and at the same time fully God. God, living everyday life with ordinary people—fishermen, tax collectors, mothers and children, even prostitutes—is the amazing center of this story. Historian of religion Mircea Eliade says, "Since God was *incarnated*, that is, since he took on a *historically conditioned human existence*, history acquires the possibility of being sanctified. . . . For God's interventions in history, and above all his incarnation in the historical person of Jesus Christ, have a transhistorical purpose—*the salvation* of man."[23] God was working within the ordinary events of life to fulfill his purposes.

Jesus lived about thirty-three years. During his public ministry, which was only three years long, he gathered about him a small group of followers, preparing them to continue his ministry after he left. During those three years Jesus inaugurated the kingdom of heaven, promising that it would grow from a tiny seed into a large tree (Mt 13:31-32). His kingdom does not exist in a geographical location; it is within those who have come under God's rule. Jesus taught that we enter God's kingdom by spiritual birth, not physical birth (Jn 3:1-16). He claimed to be the only means of entry. "I am the way, the truth, and the life. No one comes to the Father except through me," he said (Jn 14:6). But the invitation for citizenship is extended to all peoples (Mt 28:18).

Most new nations come to birth through war and public declarations. But the heavenly kingdom came through weakness and death, not through an army of angels. It was Christ's death on the cross, a shameful Roman execution, that rescued us from our sins. He was vindicated when he "was raised on the third day" (1 Cor 15:3). Unlike gods in other religions who live in a mythical realm, Christ died a physical death and was raised bodily from the tomb. Forty days after his death and resurrection he returned to heaven. Now he rules over all things—the past, the present and the future. One day he will return with the armies of heaven to rule as a powerful king (Eph 1:20-23).

Living in the Extended "Third Chapter" of God's Story
We can think of the biblical story as being told in four chapters: (1) creation, (2) rebellion and sin, (3) redemption and (4) new creation. Actually, chapters two and three overlap, and chapters three and four run parallel for awhile. But eventually chapter four, the new creation, will be the full resolution of this age-long story. The rebellion and sin of the second chapter will be over and the redemption of chapter three will completed. It is to this third chapter, where sin and rebellion, redemption and the beginnings of the new creation are being played out all together, that we now turn—the extended and complex third chapter.

The church as Christ's body on earth keeps and tells the story. Those who respond to Christ's call are his disciples. He told his followers, "You did not choose me but I chose you. And I appointed you to go and bear fruit, fruit that will last" (Jn 15:16). Practical actions of care are "bearing fruit." They are signs of our faith in the end of the story. John, the writer of the book of Revelation, heard these words from heaven: "Death will be no more: mourning and crying and pain will be no more" (Rev 21:4). The sure hope that one day God himself will heal creation has inspired Christians through the ages to work in hope. Christian nurses are participants in God's story.

Today, as nurses take up our roles in God's story, Jesus is still with us (Mt 28:20). After his ascension he poured out his Spirit, enabling his followers to bear witness to him by word and deed. Peter explained to an amazed crowd at the first Pentecost: "This Jesus God raised up, and of that all of us are witnesses. Being therefore exalted at the right hand of God, and having received from the Father the promise of the Holy Spirit, he has poured out this that you both see and hear" (Acts 2:32-33). After healing a crippled man a few days later, Peter explained to puzzled religious leaders that it was the name of Jesus that had healed the man (Acts 3:15-16).

The presence of Jesus enables Christian nurses to persevere in hope in very difficult circumstances. His Spirit guides us as we respond to him. It was the Spirit of Jesus who urged Elaine to talk to Mary Ann in the opening story. Elaine could not assure Mary Ann that her husband would return. She was not even certain how her own marriage would work out. Elaine offered the hope of God's presence instead.

We might ask, "So what good is believing God's story if we may not get what we desperately need or want?" People sometimes answer this question by glibly saying that everything works out for the best in the end. But these words are not true. Awful things usually lead to awful results. For example, abused children often become abusers themselves.

What then is a better response? The apostle Paul wrote to Christians suffering for their faith: "We know that all things work together for good for those who love God, who are called according to his purpose" (Rom 8:28). These words, often spoken as bland and useless assurance, are addressed to lovers of God, members of his kingdom. The promised good is God's long-term purpose and not necessarily our immediate desires. The goal of God's story is creating a new humanity, new people who love him. God is working in his people making them like Jesus Christ (Rom 8:29). So the good that God brings out of bad things comes when he uses them to make us like Jesus. That may take a long time. Jesus said our first goal in life should be to seek the kingdom of God and his righteousness (Mt 6:33). What we should fear most is losing our souls, not our lives (Mt 10:28).

But God is not concerned only with his long-term goal for us. He suffers with those who have chronic pain. He grieves with the mother whose child is dying. He wants the wonderful processes that heal our bodies to work. Jesus said, "Are not two sparrows sold for a penny? Yet not one of them will fall to the ground apart from your Father. And even the hairs of our head are all counted. So do not be afraid; you are of more value than many sparrows" (Mt 10:29-30).

What Elaine can promise Mary Ann is that nothing can separate her from the love of God, not even the breakup of her marriage. Nothing that happens must cause us to lose our souls. Nothing can make Jesus turn away from us. His loving presence is constant (Rom 8:39).

Christians have found hope in this assurance through the centuries. This is the hope that will sustain nurses in the changing health care system. This is the hope that we can offer our patients when all other hopes are lost.

Hopeful Living in Hard Times

When Jesus' disciples asked him about the future, he told them that the dates and times of future events were not for them to know. They were to simply get on with the tasks at hand, trusting God for direction and empowerment. They were to be witnesses for Jesus wherever they lived and worked (Acts 1:6-8). Jesus himself modeled this almost casual attitude toward life. He did not schedule his activities as modern people do. He went from place to place seemingly without preplanning. He was open to the interruptions of individuals along the way—people like blind beggars, untouchable lepers, mothers with children to bless.

Yet there was a consistency to his life that reflected his mission. He left one place after healing many when still more were gathering to see him. "Let us go on the neighboring towns, so that I may proclaim the message there also; for that is what I came to do" (Mk 1:38). He did speak often of going to Jerusalem and predicted that he would be captured, executed and then vindicated. Jesus possessed an inner coordination and purpose that directed his life. He was not driven to achieve a goal, yet he moved steadfastly toward what he knew the Father had in store for him. The unity of his life sprang from his understanding of the way in which God carries out his purposes.

Living in God's true story, learning how he works out his purposes, trusting when we can't see him working; these all enable nurses to live in hope. We want to bear this hope to patients and colleagues (Eph 1:20-23). We do not need to merely "hope in hope." We know the God of hope who fills us with peace and joy in believing, so that we may abound in hope by the power of the Holy Spirit (Rom 15:13).

Phyllis Karns is one such bearer of hope. She tells the story of Joanne, a thirty-five-year-old woman with a terminal illness. Joanne's greatest concern was for the care of her children after her death.

Phyllis showed her two instances in the Bible where mothers gave their children over to be cared for by others in less than ideal situations. One was Hannah, mother of the prophet Samuel, who allowed him to be raised in the household of a corrupted priesthood (1 Sam 1:24-28). The other was Moses' mother, Jocebed, who gave her son to be raised by a heathen princess in a climate of wealth, power and pagan religion (Ex 2). Each of the mothers was willing to trust God to be faithful in overseeing the growth and development of her child and to accept that God truly loved and would take care of the child.

Phyllis prayed with the dying mother, who was able to trust Jesus as Lord of the future for her children as well as for her own life after her death.[24]

Story As a Way of Knowing

We have focused thus far on living in God's story as the only way to find the hope so important in nursing. But story is also a way of knowing, a way of discovering truth. Nurse educator Patricia Benner writes of the power of story for nursing as ethical practice.[25] Theologian Stanley Hauerwas argues that narrative is central to explain the truth of Christian life both for learning our identity and for learning moral truth.[26]

Stories give content to moral words like love and justice, courage and temperance. But how do we know when stories are true stories, not necessarily true in the sense that they actually happened but true in the sense that they tell us right things? For example, if we tell a story about "good" nursing care where a nurse refused a patient's request that would lead to her or his death, how can we know that it is truly good? Perhaps another nurse telling the story would label it bad care, saying that the patient's wishes should have been followed.

It is God's story that shows us the way. We continually test the smaller stories of our lives against his story. How do they fit within it? Do they continue to tell God's story, or do they belong to another story of sin and rebellion? The amazing thing is that God actually invites us to help tell his story by our lives.

God's story also teaches us who we are: historical beings dependent on God and others. We often introduce ourselves by telling the story of our lives. However, it is not only others who learn to know us by our stories; we learn to know ourselves. Many fearful nursing students have been amazed to discover that they actually knew more than they thought about patient care. Likewise, patients who trembled at the prospect of a painful treatment have come through amazed at their own strength. This is why telling stories to children and adults can be a powerful source of encouragement.

Because God is telling his story in our environment, we can have hope, we can know ourselves, and we can know moral truth. The key for nurses is to live within his story and to tell it to ourselves and each other over and over. To learn it well.

Part Four

Health as the
Goal of Nursing

10

Working
Toward *Shalom*

SUSAN STOOD ON MY (JUDY'S) DOORSTEP, A GLOWING PICTURE of health. Her eyes flashed with enthusiasm for life, and a deep sense of joy radiated from her face, but the large mass on her neck betrayed another force at work in her body. Susan was on her way home from radiation therapy for a rapidly growing thyroid cancer, but she had never felt more alive.

She wanted to tell me how much her relationship with God and the friendships she had developed within the congregation meant to her, and how that gave her a different perspective on her illness. She knew she was dying, but she felt at peace. She was ready to meet God, and she knew that her husband, Joe, would not be left alone—people in the church would continue to care for him.

Susan's view of the church had not always been this positive. As a young woman, Susan and Joe were active church members in a neighboring congregation. She raised her family in a Christian home and taught Sunday school for several years. However, after her daughters were confirmed they gradually drifted away from the church. When her oldest daughter became engaged, she called the pastor asking him to officiate at her wedding. The pastor refused, stating that since she was no longer an active member, it was against his policy to perform the ceremony for her. The incident hurt Susan deeply. She grew angry and bitter toward God and the church. She and Joe withdrew from the congregation and did not participate in any church activities for about twenty years.

During those years away from their church, Joe passed our church building every Sunday morning on his way to the golf course. Each time, he felt something drawing him into the building. Finally he began attending worship, then joined a Sunday-school class, where he once again began to grow in his faith and delighted in the fellowship with people in the church. For years the Sunday-school class prayed with him that Susan would release her bitterness and return to church with him. She slipped in occasionally but kept her distance. Then tragedies began to strike. First a son-in-law died in an automobile accident. Then Susan's brother died of a rapid-growing thyroid cancer. Within months Susan faced the same diagnosis.

Throughout all the crises, the church ministered to Susan through notes, visits, flowers and prayers. Finally her resistance broke down. She came back into a vital faith and began to enjoy the fellowship of the community of God's people.

As Susan's illness progressed and she became homebound, I visited her as a volunteer parish nurse. We discussed the importance of taking her pain medication and why she didn't have to worry about becoming addicted. We developed a strategy to deal with the side effects of her medication. Our primary focus, though, was on her relationships: with her husband, her family, the church community and God. We prayed together, wept and hugged. Susan died just before Christmas. Her funeral was a celebration of life and faith—a testimony to the health God offers us in his *shalom*.

What Is Health?

The popular media portray health as youthful appearance, hard muscles, sleek bodies, clear skin and cavity-free teeth. Nursing literature is increasingly moving to the other extreme. Health is "expanding consciousness," according to nursing theorist Margaret Newman.[1] It is "essentially synonymous with *becoming*, which is an open, rhythmically coconstituting process of the human-universe interrelationship," according to theorist Rosemarie Parse.[2]

One nursing text compiled the current definitions of health and listed these:

□ a dynamic process
□ determined subjectively and objectively
□ a goal
□ being able to take care of yourself
□ optimal functioning in body, mind and spirit
□ integrity of self
□ a sense of wholeness
□ coping adaptively
□ a subjective experience
□ growing and becoming
□ a broad concept[3]

According to current nursing literature, health is indeed a broad concept; so broad, in fact, that it ceases to be an adequate goal for nursing. Margaret Newman even states, "Health encompasses conditions that heretofore were described as illness, or in medical terms, pathology."[4] For the most part, contemporary nursing definitions of health focus primarily on a state of mind. Older definitions and conventional wisdom (as represented by television commercials) focus on the body. The World Health Organization (WHO) idealistically defined health in 1946 as "a state of complete physical, mental, and social well-being and not merely the absence of disease or infirmity." It was a definition that medical ethicist Daniel Callahan says set the stage for a conception of health that literally encompasses every element of human happiness.[5]

Earlier I said that Susan radiated health despite her tumor. She obviously did not meet the WHO standard of health. On what basis could I say that Susan was "healthy"? What is the difference between that understanding of health and Margaret Newman's? Susan demonstrated health in her attitudes and relationships, but the tumor itself was not encompassed in her health—it remained a very serious pathology. However, if we view the person as an integrated whole, created to live in harmony with God, self, others and the environment,[6] then health means being able to function as God created us to be. It involves reconciliation with God and others, forgiving and accepting forgiveness, loving and being loved, finding meaning and purpose in life leading to a sense of joy and hope, as well as freedom from physical ailments.

Health Is Culturally Defined

To some extent health is culturally understood. Nursing theorist Madeleine Leininger explains, "Our rapidly growing multicultural world makes it imperative that nurses understand different cultures to work and function effectively with people having different values, beliefs, and ideas about nursing, health, caring, wellness, illness, death, and disabilities."[7] She sees human caring as the heart of nursing and as a universal phenomenon. "*Health* refers to a state of well-being that is culturally defined, valued, and practiced, and which reflects the ability of individuals (or groups) to perform their daily role activities in culturally expressed, beneficial, and patterned lifeways."[8] Hence nurses must draw their goals for nursing from the persons or groups in their care.

Biblical anthropologists Bruce Malina and Richard Rohrbaugh attempt to uncover the cultural understanding of health found in the time of Jesus.[9] They stress that in ancient Mediterranean culture a person's state of being was more important than the ability to act or function.

> Illness is not so much a biomedical matter as it is a social one. It is attributed to social causes, not physical ones. Because sin is a breach of interpersonal relationship, sin and sickness go together. Illness is not so much a medical matter as a matter of deviance from the cultural norms and values.[10]

Malina and Rohrbaugh view Jesus' healings primarily as restoring the person to the worshiping community. Healing is directly related to the cultural belief system.

Missionary physician Tony Atkins describes the African view of health in a similar way, as a function of community. He explains, "It is an indigenous concept that acceptance within, and harmony with, family and society are important elements in healing and preserving the health of people."[11] He compares the African view to the biblical understanding of health and concludes, "For the Jew, as for many people in tribal societies today, health was essentially a positive quality that derived from the fact that people existed in total harmony with the world and in harmony with God."[12]

A Biblical Understanding of Health

The biblical understanding of health is closely related to the concept of *shalom.* Often translated as *peace, shalom* actually incorporates all the elements that go into making a God-centered community—peace, prosperity, rest, safety, security, justice, happiness, health, welfare, wholeness. Christian philosopher Nicholas Wolterstorff defines *shalom* as "the human being dwelling at peace in all his or her relationships: with God, with self, with fellows, with nature."[13] The future new Jerusalem described in Revelation 21:2-4 illustrates the meaning of *shalom:*

> And I saw the holy city, the new Jerusalem, coming down out of heaven from God, prepared as a bride adorned for her husband. And I heard a loud voice from the throne saying, "See, the home of God is among mortals. He will dwell with them as their God; they will be his peoples, and God himself will be with them; he will wipe every tear from their eyes. Death will be no more; mourning and crying and pain will be no more, for the first things have passed away."

Like the WHO definition, the concept of *shalom* is too broad to be the goal of nursing, but it provides a perspective through which we can frame our understanding of health. Linked to the biblical understanding of the person, *shalom* points us to how the healthy person functions. It includes the physical, psychosocial and spiritual dimensions of the person.

The late theologian Paul Tillich illuminates the idea of *dimensions* by saying that the person should not be considered "as a composite of several levels, such as body, soul, spirit, but as a multidimensional unity." The dimensions do not "lie alongside, but within each other."[14] He then describes six dimensions: mechanical, chemical, biological, psychological, spiritual and historical. He proposes that health cannot be defined apart from its opposite—disease—and disease affects all dimensions of the person. True healing takes place only when all six dimensions are healthy; however, in this life we must usually be content with limited healing. Ultimate healing comes through Jesus Christ, who is the *sōtēr*—a Greek term that means both *savior* and *healer.*

The interrelationship between health and salvation in the New Testament is striking. When a group of men brought their paralyzed friend to Jesus, they were surprised to hear Jesus say to him, "Your sins are forgiven" (Mk 2:5; Lk 5:20). He then went on to heal him physically. There seems to have been a relationship between the man's need for forgiveness and his illness. When a woman with chronic vaginal bleeding touched the hem of Jesus' garment, he replied to her, "Your faith has made you well," implying a relationship between faith and healing (Mt 9:21).

The Greek word *sōzō,* used here and elsewhere for *healing* (see Mk 5:23; 6:56; 10:52; Lk 8:48-50; 17:19; 18:42; Acts 4:9; 14:9; Jas 5:15) is translated in other passages as *salvation* (see, for example, Mt 1:21; 10:22; 19:25; 24:22; Mk 16:16; Lk 13:23-24; Jn 3:17; 10:9; Acts 2:21; 4:12; 11:14; Rom 10:9). When Jesus cleansed the ten lepers (Lk 17:11-19), only one returned to thank him. Jesus told that man, "Your faith has made you well *(sōzō)*." All ten were cleansed of leprosy, but only the one who returned found complete healing—and it was intimately wrapped up in his ability to praise God. The whole point of Jesus' healing people was to restore them to a fuller, richer relationship with God and the faith community.

Theologian Jürgen Moltmann explains:

> Healing consists of the restoration of disrupted community, and the sharing and communication of life. Jesus heals the sick by restoring their fellowship with God.[15]

Theologian Thomas Droege expands this idea:

> Since wholeness is more than physical well-being, the healings of Jesus also effected changes in the meanings and values of those whom he encountered. Jesus consistently called people to repentance. He invited people to turn away from those things that brought division and disintegration into their lives and to become responsible for their own

health as well as the health of others.[16]

Such a definition goes far beyond the scope of nursing, but it also reveals something of our relationship to other members of the health care team and to the Christian community. Because people are multidimensional beings in need of holistic healing, we are also a multidimensional healing community. Nursing encompasses only one dimension of health care. However, the role of the nurse does not necessarily "lie alongside" medicine and pastoral care; in many ways it is "within" both. It involves recognition that both the nurse and the person receiving care are members of a community and dependent upon God. Healing requires us to function harmoniously within those communities and in partnership with God.

Implications for Nursing Practice

Functioning under such definitions leads to some fuzzy distinctions, but it acknowledges what we already know and reduces the spirit of competition. There will be times when nursing stretches to include practicing medicine. Nurses in developing countries with scarce resources and few physicians have always gone far beyond the limits of traditional nursing—diagnosing, treating, prescribing, and even performing surgery.[17] Today's advanced practice roles also push hard into the once iron-clad bounds of medicine.[18] In a similar way, nursing borders on entering into the role of clergy—even to the point of organizing through religious orders or working as parish nurses and deacon nurses on churches' ministerial staffs. Rather than fight turf battles, we need to recognize that the pursuit of health must remain multidimensional and interdisciplinary. Just when we think we have the lines drawn properly they will shift again.

What then are the implications of this multidimensional understanding of health for nursing? Florence Nightingale understood nursing to be taking "personal charge of the health of others."[19] If we are to take charge of it, we must know what it is!

Nurse educator Ruth Stoll defines health as having five dimensions:

Wholeness. Health is wholeness, the harmonious unity of the person within himself and outwardly with God and her/his environment.

Transformation. Health is a dynamic process of internal transformations progressively reflected in the person's outward behavior.

Relationship. Health is the experiencing of loving, just and forgiving relationships with God, self and others that provides meaning and purpose in life.

Coping and adaptation. Health is a reality-oriented perspective that allows the person to adapt and cope with internal and external change and stress.

Human paradox. Health is creative living with the human paradox of being and becoming, of living with sin, redemption and restoration.[20]

Theologian Karl Barth defined health simply as "the power to be as man exercised in the powers of the vital functions of soul and body."[21] In other words, it is to be all that God created us to be. Missionary physician Daniel Fountain cautions:

> Health cannot be defined. It is not simply an object for analysis. To render it such is to think secularly about health. Health is life, a gift we receive, an endowment we are to develop, and a journey we are to pursue. We can observe and analyze much along the way. We can manipulate and improve certain aspects of health and life. But we can never comprehend the whole.[22]

While it may be true that we can never fully grasp the concept of health (hence the wide range of definitions), most people instinctively know what it means to be healthy. Perhaps Tillich's insistence that health can be defined only in contrast to its opposite—disease—can help direct our understanding. People all over the world, in every culture, seek health care when pain or disability prevents them from attending to the activities of daily living. What are they hoping to find? At first they are looking for relief from pain, ability to function, and restoration to their social environment. This level is primarily physical. Beyond that, people may seek to eliminate the underlying causes of the immediate problem. At this level the psychosocial and spiritual dimensions enter into the health care spectrum.

When our operational definition of health neglects the physical dimension, nurses can justify avoiding the hard—and often unpleasant—work of caring for the body. We also eliminate the primary motivation most people have for seeking health care. Pain, nausea, fever and conditions that limit our ability to work and play drive us to seek help.

God created us with bodies. The physical is real. It is not an illusion. Regardless of how strongly certain nursing theorists may argue that the biological functions are illusory and can be controlled by the mind, our bodies are still subject to injury and illness. We have only to stub a toe to be convinced. While the mind certainly has a great deal to do with wellness and healing, disease is real. Bacteria and viruses can invade even the strongest immune system. Cancer and heart disease afflict the most ardent health enthusiast.

The physical dimension certainly dominates most people's thinking about health. Daniel Callahan suggests that the best definition for health might be "a state of physical well-being."[23] But that definition will not satisfy today's nursing theorists—or the biblical concept of *shalom.*

Our definition of health must also include the psychosocial and spiritual dimensions. It is here that New Paradigm thought has stepped into the gap left by our overdependence upon the scientific "medical model" of health care. New Paradigm holistic health care strikes a chord in people who have been conditioned by our modernist culture to expect that every physical problem can be "fixed." They turn to alternative therapies when scientific medicine does not work completely, results in unpleasant side effects or proves exorbitantly expensive. One of the primary drawing points of these alternative therapies is the emphasis they place on personal control, as well as their appeal to ancient spiritual wisdom.

In the early 1960s physician Halbert Dunn began talking about "high level wellness,"[24] which set the stage for viewing health as an individual achievement that can be controlled by the mind. There is a great deal of truth to this concept. Every nurse can relate stories of people who overcame great odds to recover rapidly because of sheer will power, or others who died when they lost hope. But the mortality rate remains 100 percent. In fact, if one compares life expectancy in populations where alternative therapies are commonly practiced (such as in China or India) with others where allo-pathic medicine prevails, the numbers are tilted greatly in favor of Western medicine.

A Christian view of health must also incorporate a realistic under-standing of human suffering and mortality and the hope of eternal life. There are forces at work in the world that we cannot fully control, even with science or mind control—microorganisms, genetics, environmental pollut-ants, violence, accidents, spiritual influences. We are not God. We will eventually get sick and die. To view health as *shalom* means to stand with those who are sick and dying and to encompass them in the fellowship of the Christian community and the presence of God.

Putting Health in a Larger Context

The Christian, then, places health within a larger context. It can be a radiant health in the midst of terrible physical disability. Conversely, health can be absent in a person with a well-toned body. Health usually shows itself as "a state of physical well-being,"[25] but ultimately it is *shalom*, a God-centered wholeness that enables the person to live in harmony with self, God, others and the environment.

Medical ethicists Stephen Lammers and Allen Verhey assert, "Defini-tions of health turn out to be important because in doing the defining, we must explore the relationship of health to other human goods; the relation-ship of health and responsibility, both of individuals and of the medical [or nursing] profession; and the relationship of health and those conventional modes of treating and coping with illness."[26] So how does health shape our goals for nursing?

Let's go back to Susan, my radiantly healthy dying friend. As a nurse I acknowledged the value of expert scientific medical care and dealt with her physical condition. At the same time, as a parish nurse I represented the caring Christian community and worked toward a different kind of health. During those months before she died, Susan was surrounded by family, friends and a Christian community that included her visiting nurses. Together we had worked toward *shalom*.

Health is essentially living according to God's purposes, even in the face of suffering and death. It includes the physical dimension; therefore, we work toward maintaining optimal physical function and providing comfort measures. However, complete health also means living in harmonious relationship with God and our neighbors; therefore, nursing also includes assisting patients in establishing and maintaining a relationship with God through Jesus Christ, as well as facilitating healing relationships among people.

A final example illustrates this kind of health. Recently, my (Judy's) phone rang. A weak voice mumbled slowly, "I . . . can't . . . take it! I'm . . . I'm . . . going to . . . commit . . . suicide."

George was an old friend. I recognized his voice immediately. Cancer had been slowly robbing him of life over the past ten years. His wife, Anna, had died a year before. He lived alone now. A month earlier he had been admitted to the hospital five times for various complications, then transferred to a nursing home, where he refused to stay.

"Have you taken anything you shouldn't?" I asked, fearing the worst.

"No, I'm too scared. But you said to call if I ever felt this way, and I do."

I dropped everything and drove to his house. Knowing George was a hunter, with guns in the house as well as pills, I feared what I might find. When I arrived, George was sitting in a recliner looking dejected, surrounded by boxes of gastrostomy feedings, bottles of pills and medical equipment. He grabbed my hands and poured out his feelings of agony. I listened, then prayed for him, taking his concerns to the Lord. Then he rose out of his chair, fell on his face sobbing, and pleaded with the Lord himself. A short time later, while we were talking, his brother arrived.

Jake asked George how he was doing. George looked at me and said, "You tell him." We talked about his suicidal feelings and discussed options. Jake settled into the other chair. Assured that George was in good hands for the time being, I left.

George is a broken man. However, the brokenness has come not so much from his cancer as from his aloneness. As long as Anna was with him, he faced the repeated surgeries and painful procedures with a good sense of optimism and strength. Even after Anna died, George seemed to do pretty well as long as he could come out to the healing services at church. But now he was alone, isolated in his home despite occasional visits from friends, family and the visiting nurse. He felt as if God had left him as well.

Although talk of individualism, self-care and autonomy falls easily from our tongues today, God made us for community. Healing—*wholeness*—comes only in community, not in self-actualization or radical autonomy. Wholeness is not an achievement, something we can accomplish. It is a gift from God and a way of living in community.

How can we bring *wholeness* to those in our care? First, we offer everything in our nursing knowledge and skill to bring comfort and healing. The visiting nurse came the next day to care for George's physical needs. She called his physician to get his pain and anxiety medication adjusted, and she revised his feeding schedule. But Christian nursing can't stop there. We give ourselves, as members of the body of Christ, to draw our patients into a community of caring. For George, that community went to work, planning follow-up visits, prayer calls and other supportive measures. Ultimately, though, his wholeness will come through being reconciled to God.

By the next evening George was surrounded by friends and family. His sister called to say she would come and stay with him for two weeks. His pain and anxiety were under control. He no longer felt like committing suicide. In his words, "It was the difference between night and day."

What changed George's condition? The prayer? The physical interventions? The presence and support of a caring community? All of the above. George is still a very sick man—terminally ill—but he is experiencing health in a new way. He is living in *shalom*.

11

Hope in Suffering

IN A MOMENT OF DESPAIR, JOE COLLINS TOOK A SHOTGUN, placed it in his mouth and pulled the trigger. He intended to blow his brains out. Instead, he lost half his face. All that remained was one bulging eye, two holes where his nose should have been and a mouth opening only big enough to hold the cigarette that constantly dangled from his lips. A heavy cloud of gloom hung over his head.

Joe Collins was my (Judy's) first patient. Our assignment was to "talk to patients." But Joe couldn't talk; he merely grunted occasionally. He was faced with extensive reconstructive surgery to give him back the life he didn't want to live. Joe's suffering overwhelmed me. I could not even look at him, much less carry on a conversation. I made his bed, scrubbed his bedside table until it shined, filled his water pitcher and tried to ask a few questions he could answer with a grunt.

The age-old question *How can a just and loving God allow people to suffer?* confronts every nursing student as soon as clinical experience begins. Theologians call this question *theodicy.* Although Joe's physical suffering was self-inflicted, many other cases followed that were harder to understand—a twenty-three-year-old mother of a newborn, dying of ovarian cancer; a pediatric unit filled with hydrocephalic infants and toddlers dying of leukemia; an esteemed former professor paralyzed and brain-damaged from a stroke.

The questions loom larger when suffering comes closer to home—your mother is suddenly stricken with a myocardial infarction; a brother is killed in an automobile accident; your position at work is dissolved, and you find yourself unemployed. No longer do you just ask, *Why?* Now you implore, *Why me?*

Several years ago, as my father-in-law sat slumped in a wheelchair after years of struggling through the effects of a series of strokes, my husband asked him, "Pop, do you ever ask God, *Why me?*" My father-in-law, a retired pastor, had spent his life in dedicated service to God and other people. He deserved a better end than this.

Pop looked at his son and, with great effort, answered, "No, the proper question is, *Why not me?*"

Suffering is a great mystery. It doesn't make sense to us. Our culture concentrates time and attention on avoiding suffering. And when it becomes impossible to eliminate the suffering, many have decided to remove the suffering person through euthanasia. Such action flies in the face of the Christian hope.

Christians certainly don't have all the answers, but we can trust the God who does. The Bible and church history give us some helpful insights into suffering—insights that do not solve the dilemma but at least make it more bearable. Interestingly, the early Christians, who suffered intense persecution and oppression, did not ask the *theodicy* question.[1] That came later, as Christians had more leisure time to spend in reflection Instead of asking *Why?*, the first-century church concentrated on supporting the sufferer (1 Pet 4:12-15; 2 Cor 8:1-2; Gal 6:2).

Our culture, on the other hand, has convinced us that we deserve what we get. That philosophy is fine as long as we are healthy, affluent and successful. But it rapidly fails when debilitating illness, unemployment or failure strikes unexpectedly. Even Christians, who trust in God's grace, may subtly assume that a person must have done something wrong to deserve the problems that come—just as Hindus believe that suffering comes from bad *karma.* That is not a Christian perspective.

The Mystery of Suffering

Suffering remains a mystery we cannot fully explain, but God has given us some hints about it, and we can summarize what we do know.

First, suffering came into the world through sin. Suffering was not part of God's original creation, but he gave us the freedom to disobey him, with suffering as a result of that disobedience (Gen 1—3). Therefore, all people, as well as all of creation, suffer (Rom 8:18-39). Although some suffering is the direct result of an individual's sin (for example, wounds from violent behavior, sexually transmitted diseases from promiscuity, addiction from substance abuse), we cannot automatically blame an individual for his or her suffering (Jn 9:1-7; Job 1—2). Most suffering comes from factors over which we have no control. Satan causes some suffering (1 Pet 5:8-9; Rev 2:10), and involvement in Christian ministry often brings suffering (2 Cor 6:4-10; 2 Tim 1:8). Suffering is part of life. We can expect it. Rather than ask "Why me?" we should wonder "Why not me?" (1 Pet 4:12-19).

Second, we can be assured that God is involved in our suffering. God lovingly walks with us in our suffering (Is 43:1-7). He suffers for us (Lk 22:1-71; 23:32-49; Heb 4:14-16). Through the death and resurrection of Jesus Christ the power of sin was broken, so that one day suffering will cease entirely (Rev 21:1-4; Is 35:1-10; 53:1-12). In the meantime, God gives us the privilege of suffering for him (Phil 1:29). He uses suffering to refine, mature us and discipline us (Is 48:9-11; Heb 12:3-13; 1 Pet 1:6-9). He demonstrates his power and love in the midst of our suffering (2 Cor 12:7-10).

Third, we can respond to suffering in faith. Our own suffering equips us to help others who suffer (2 Cor 1:3-11; Rom 5:1-5). We join together with the body of Christ, the church, to care for those who suffer either physically or spiritually (Mt 25:31-46; Lk 10:1-12; 25-37; 1 Cor 12:26).

Finally, we endure suffering with patience and hope, trusting in God's compassion and mercy (Jas 5:7-11). Although suicide or euthanasia may seem to be a way out of suffering, they are not acceptable to God (Ex 20:13; Num 11:15; Job 3:11-13; Jer 20:14-15; Phil 1:19-24). Suffering remains a mystery which cannot be fully understood or controlled (Job 1—2; 42).

Suffering in Other Religions and Belief Systems

Other religions hold different views of suffering. As nurses care for people from different religious traditions, they should be aware of some of the major views. The descriptions below are general, and a nurse caring for persons of these religions will want to do more in-depth study, as well as learn from the patients themselves. Not only do these views of suffering apply to professed adherents of other religions and cultures, but many of these ideas have become common within our culture and even permeated the understanding of some Christians.

Hinduism. In Hinduism, suffering is viewed as the result of bad *karma* or destiny created in a previous existence. In other words, the sufferer is paying for something done when he or she was another person or creature. According to the doctrine of *samsara* (transmigration) all life goes through an endless succession of rebirths. Hindus teach that the appropriate response to suffering is resignation to one's fate while, at the same time, trying to create good *karma* for one's next existence. Release and liberation from the wheel of life (*moksha* or *mukti*) comes when one realizes that his or her individual soul *(Atman)* is identical with the universal soul *(Brahman)*. The only way to finally escape suffering is to lose one's individual identity in the universal soul or the Absolute, a state of bliss called *Nirvana. Nirvana* is achieved by detachment from the finite self and attachment to reality as a whole.

The Hindu sees three basic approaches for achieving *Nirvana* or salvation. (1) Salvation by knowledge *(Jnana Yoga)* is acquired by listening to the sages and the scriptures, practicing meditation by turning awareness inward, and realizing the *Atman-Brahman* identity. (2) Salvation can come by devotion *(Bhakti Yoga)* to a particular manifestation of God (Brahma the creator, Vishnu the preserver, and Shiva the destroyer and his wife Kali), and hope to break through to a union with God. (3) Salvation by correct works *(Karma Yoga)* is gained by performing ceremonies, sacrifices, pilgrimages and other good actions without attachment of desire for their rewards. All of these methods may also include *Raja Yoga*, an involved technique of meditation which includes control over the body, breathing and thoughts.[2]

Buddhism. The Buddhist sees suffering as the result of human desire and attachment to people and things. The goal of each Buddhist is to attain *Nirvana,* a release from suffering, desire and the finite self. In *Nirvana* there is no enduring self, but a total awareness and total being leading to enlightenment. Buddhism is built on the Four Noble Truths: (1) Life is full of pain and suffering *(dukkha).* This is especially evident in birth, sickness, decay, death, and the presence of hated things and separation from loved things. Even the forces that hold life together *(skandas)* are full of suffering. These include the body, senses, thoughts, feelings and consciousness. (2) Suffering is caused by *tanha,* the desire or thirst for pleasure, existence and prosperity. (3) Suffering can be overcome by eliminating these cravings. (4) This is done by following the Eightfold Path.

The Eightfold Path is a system of therapy designed to develop habits that will release people from the restrictions caused by ignorance and craving and lead to purification of consciousness or enlightenment. It consists of: (1) right knowledge (the Four Noble Truths), (2) right aspirations (intentions), (3) right speech, (4) right conduct, (5) right livelihood (occupation), (6) right effort, (7) right mindfulness (self-analysis) and (8) right meditation.[3]

There are two main divisions of Buddhism: Greater Vehicle *(Mahayana)* Buddhism and Lesser Vehicle *(Theravada)* Buddhism, in which the ways of achieving *Nirvana* differ. In Mahayana Buddhism the ideal is to become a bodhisattva, one who concentrates on reducing the suffering of others. There is less emphasis on withdrawal and meditation and more on sacrificing oneself out of compassion for living beings. By meditating, though, the aspiring Bodhisattva realizes that nothing we see has genuine reality and that the real nature of things is empty. Meditation is seen as the way to a mystical nondualistic experience of reality in which there are no distinctions and no self.[4]

Judaism. Jews accept the reality of human suffering. The question raised in the Hebrew Bible (the Christian Old Testament) concerns the distribution of suffering: *Why do some people suffer and others not?* (Job 21:7-16; Ps 94:3-7). Why do the wicked not suffer when those who try to keep faith with God do? God is both compassionate and all-powerful, so why does this injustice occur? Suffering is sometimes explained as punishment for sin and other times as a means of testing character and faithfulness. But this does not explain all suffering. The Bible also speaks of a radical intervention by God in human affairs in which undeserved suffering will be made right by the coming of a Messiah to set up God's kingdom.[5]

Many modern Jews hold a more secular view of suffering that emphasizes the need to survive it with courage and dignity. Because of the extreme suffering throughout Jewish history, many Jews today hold that they must be strong to defend themselves against further suffering. Some of them still look forward to a coming Messiah who will lead them to freedom and peace, while others maintain that only human efforts will reach these goals.[6]

Islam. For Muslims, suffering is to be expected as a part of living. God (Allah) is viewed as all-powerful and compassionate. Because Allah is all-powerful, everything that happens, including suffering, is under his control. The proper human response is to submit to the will of Allah in all things, including suffering. Suffering is sometimes viewed as punishment for evil, but more often as a means (instrument) of developing character. In some cases voluntary suffering undertaken for God is seen as meritorious.[7] At the same time, there are social means for attacking suffering through almsgiving *(zakat)*. There is a day of judgment in which each person's deeds will be weighed on a pair of balances to determine the person's destiny. Heaven is a place of sensuous delight and gratification.

The Five Pillars of Islam are the main religious practices. They are: (1) reciting the *Shahadah,* "There is no God but Allah, and Mohammed is his prophet," aloud several times daily; (2) praying prescribed prayers *(salat)* five times a day; (3) almsgiving *(zakat);* (4) fasting during the month of Ramadan by not eating or drinking anything during the daylight hours; (5) going on a pilgrimage to Mecca *(Hajj)* at least once in a lifetime. A Muslim must also be a good spokesperson for the faith.[8]

Animism. Many people in almost every culture believe that spirits animate, or live in, all things, both the living and the inert. This folk belief may be the primary religion of its adherents, but it underlies or coexists with many other religions as well. These spirits are associated with curing, magic and witchcraft. The response to suffering in this belief system is to find ways to placate the spirits or direct their attention away from the sufferer. Such techniques include charms (magic formulas), amulets, secret potions, rituals and dances.[9]

Naturalism. For the naturalist, suffering is purely the result of natural causes. Humans suffer either because they do not yet know how to avoid the natural chain of cause and effect or because they step into the chain by their own poor choices. The response to suffering is to learn how to get control of the natural chain of events through science. When that is not possible, some advocate taking control of one's own death to eliminate suffering.[10]

New Age. New Age spirituality usually sees suffering as the result of wrong thinking (imperfect consciousness) or unnecessary commitment to other people or material concerns. New Age philosophy draws from many traditions and religions, but especially from Westernized and romanticized Hinduism, Buddhism, Taoism and Theosophy. *Monism* (the belief that all is one) usually surfaces as the most central belief. New Age philosophy decries dualistic thinking for separating the creature from the Creator, good from evil, the seen from the unseen and matter from spirit. Self is viewed as the prime reality, so that as human beings expand their consciousness, they can transform themselves. Barbara Blattner, in her text *Holistic Nursing,* states: "People are responsible for their own bodies and minds. They can choose sickness or health. They have control over their lives and minds, their bodies, and their health."[11] Hence, people who suffer have chosen to do so.

New Age techniques for relieving suffering are drawn from energy manipulation and mind control, which are based on a monistic worldview. They may also use occult practices, attempting to control and manipulate the spiritual world. Many New Age thinkers appeal to Jungian psychology and quantum physics for explanations of the efficacy of their modalities.[12] Since they believe that dualistic thinking overburdens people with guilt and stress, various psychological techniques are used to rid them of guilt feelings. However, because they see no distinction between life and death, pain and happiness, assisted suicide becomes an option for ending suffering.

Searching for Healing Techniques

What, then, can we do to relieve suffering? Are any alternative therapies "safe"? Can we incorporate into our nursing care practices based on other religions? Jesus admonished his disciples to be "wise as serpents and innocent as doves" (Mt 10:16). As Christians practicing in a pluralistic health care system, we need to heed his advice. Every new technique must be carefully evaluated, not only for its effectiveness but also for its philosophical underpinnings (see appendix for guidelines). At the same time, we can trust God to protect us from being unknowingly led astray.

Some Christians believe that they can use certain alternative techniques by adapting them to a Christian understanding of their effectiveness. Others adamantly shun all practices that have any hint of Eastern or occult roots. At times we need to humbly agree to disagree when strong differences of opinion occur among Christians regarding holistic techniques. However, we are still responsible before God to be both wise and faithful. While some alternative therapies are just basic common sense—good nutrition, rest, relaxation, human touch—many of these therapies can lead those who practice them into idolatry.

Suffering often drives people to turn to alternative therapies out of desperation. They are willing to try anything, and sometimes the techniques *do* seem to bring temporary comfort. Christians may let down their guard when they see patients respond positively to various complementary approaches. Psychologist Elizabeth Hillstrom provides some helpful insights into why these therapies appear to work.[13]

First, they may be conferring actual physical benefits in ways that are not yet apparent to scientific inquiry. Research has shown real physical benefits of some herbal remedies, acupuncture and acupressure. It has not been able to demonstrate *why* they work, but it does suggest, for example, that these therapies may cause the body to release endorphins. Some alternative therapies may also bring real physical improvements indirectly through reducing stress and giving hope, love and a sense of meaning and empowerment.

In many cases, people attribute healing to alternative therapies when it is actually due to the body's ability to heal itself. Hillstrom quotes doctors as saying that 80 percent of physical ailments they treat would resolve themselves without treatment. Some benefits from holistic treatments can be attributed to placebo effect. Placebo effect has an actual physiological basis. It causes the body to produce endorphins which reduce pain and worry, allowing the immune system to function more effectively. The beneficial effects of emotional support and the communication of caring and concern can also aid in healing.

If these were the only effects of alternative therapies, we could easily incorporate them into Christian nursing. However, there are problems involved. Some apparent healings are fraudulent and trick people into thinking they are healed. This can have devastating effects when the "healed" person stops taking essential medication or discontinues life-sustaining medical care. Furthermore, many holistic alternative therapies turn to occult spiritual beings for their power. Hillstrom warns that participating in these activities may well be flirting with the demonic, and we must keep in mind that God has strictly forbidden seeking help from the spirit realm.[14]

Finding Hope in Suffering

Instead of looking to esoteric fads for healing techniques, we have a wealth of resources in our Christian heritage to bring comfort and healing to those who are suffering. Physician David Larson cites numerous research studies to document that "not only can religious beliefs help patients to cope with their illness, but a patient's religious commitment has also been found to be associated with improved clinical status and outcomes."[15] In fact, regular church attendance turned out to be a significant factor in maintaining lower blood pressure rates in twenty studies conducted over thirty years.[16] Corporate worship, prayer and studying the Bible have been shown to positively affect both physical and mental health.[17]

Sister Rosemary Donley outlines three distinct approaches to suffering within the Christian tradition. Interestingly, these approaches have become the heart of nursing from its beginning, and are second nature to most nurses.

The first spiritual response is compassionate accompaniment. . . . The compassionate person need not offer meaning or alleviation. Rather the "other" offers a quiet sharing of the experience and helps the person to sustain the burden of the suffering. . . . They are motivated by the belief that, through their presence, the suffering person may experience the presence of the Lord from whom nothing can separate us . . .

To search for meaning of personal and communal suffering is a second type of spiritual response. . . . When suffering is endowed with the glorious role of bringing a person closer to God, the person experiences relief even when the suffering itself remains. . . .

The third, and perhaps most dramatic expression of a Christian response to suffering, is action to remove the suffering itself. . . . However when a Christian response is reduced *exclusively* to action to remove suffering, there is a profound loss.[18]

The Christian tradition does not emphasize one approach to suffering over the others, so that our task becomes determining the appropriate balance between technological intervention, "meaning giving" and compassionate presence. Donley continues, "Perhaps the ordering that makes most sense in our highly technical environment is an integration of action to remove suffering and its causes with compassionate presence and meaning giving."[19] This results in nursing care that respects the person as reflecting the image of God. Physical healing is an integral dimension of the salvation offered to us through Jesus Christ.

The gospel gives us a clear mandate to provide excellent physical care, but we need not desperately seek a cure for every terminal illness or attempt to preserve biological function at any cost. Sometimes people experience healing in this life; sometimes they find it in the life to come. Christian faith gives us the perspective to realize that life is a gift from God—it is in his hands. This perspective also prevents that sense of hopelessness that sees assisted suicide as an option. However, there does come a time when chemotherapy can stop, when resuscitation efforts are futile and invasive procedures no longer help.

At that point we still have something we can *do*. Christian nurses continue to offer hope in the face of suffering and death through compassionate presence and meaning giving. Such intervention is not an *imposing* of personal beliefs on a vulnerable patient, a concern expressed by many nurses. There is no sense of manipulative proselytizing, but simply sharing the good news of Jesus Christ.

For the Christian a vital relationship with God gives strength not only to the suffering person but also to the nurse who provides that compassionate accompaniment and meaning giving. When we find ourselves looking for quick fixes for suffering, whether in technology, alternative therapies or "assistance-in-dying," we need to pull back and examine our faith commitment. Sometimes we gain the faith and strength to care for others through our own experiences of God's faithfulness in suffering.

Learning from Experience

It doesn't take long before we learn that the Lord does not allow us to profess understanding without giving us firsthand experience. The prophet Jeremiah spent time in a cistern, the apostle Paul ended up in prison, Jesus went to the cross. The truth of Romans 5:3-5 echoes throughout the pages of Scripture and into our own lives.

> We rejoice in our sufferings, knowing that suffering produces endurance, endurance produces character, and character produces hope, and hope does not disappoint us, because God's love has been poured into our hearts through the Holy Spirit which has been given to us.

There are no shortcuts to hope.

Several years ago I (Judy) experienced the confusing specter of the health care system from the other side. As I faced a series of painful procedures, major surgery and the strong possibility of cancer, powerful emotions stormed my physical and spiritual being. And I, the strong and rational one who cares for others, fell apart.

Suddenly I found myself surrounded by the remarkably supportive community of the body of Christ. People began to pray. Friends called and prayed over the phone. Colleagues stepped in without hesitation to fulfill responsibilities I couldn't handle.

In the meantime I began to cry out to the Lord. I felt guilty that I was so scared. Where was my faith? Amazingly, no one else asked that question. They just let me express my fears, listened and cared. Each morning I would awaken around four o'clock, tormented by the what-ifs. My devotional times stretched to two hours. I would begin reading the Bible, fixating in Psalm 16, pouring out my fears to the Lord, then promptly fall asleep. I would then awaken feeling at peace. It was as if I were curling up in the lap of my heavenly Father, realizing that whatever happened, he would be with me and in control.

Gradually, I began to see the good gifts of the Lord in the midst of my anxiety. Delays with tests and procedures, which at first seemed frustrating, provided time and opportunities to grow and experience the love and support of caring Christians. A visit from one friend, a Christian nurse, was a particular turning point. She asked me, "Are you afraid of dying? If so, we can talk about it." And as we talked, the fears began to lift. Suffering was beginning to produce endurance.

The object of my hope began to shift. No longer was I caught up in the immediate worries about the surgery and possible diagnosis, or even the practical concerns of whether I would live to see my children grow up, but a deep sense of the Lord's love enveloped me. When the fears began to well up again, the words of the hymn "God Will Take Care of You" began to drift through my head. Tears flowed as I realized the truth of those words. Even if I did have cancer, God would take care of me, my family and all the pressing projects that made me feel indispensable. That realization began to free me from the bondage of fear, so I could begin to reach out again to other people in their needs and get on with the work at hand. Endurance began to produce character, making me more compassionate and understanding of others who suffer.

Throughout this process I began to see the reality of the hope we have in Jesus Christ—the hope which will not disappoint us. I experienced the power of God's love being poured out through the Holy Spirit through precious times of prayer, through a deepening love for God's Word, and through the overwhelming care and support of his people. I gained a new appreciation for the body of Christ and the important role that we have as Christian nurses to provide that compassionate presence and meaning in suffering.

Instilling hope is the heart of Christian nursing. Technical competence is extremely important, but to those who are suffering and afraid, the absolute fact of Jesus Christ's death and resurrection to restore us to relationship with God holds ultimate weight. That is not an abstract theological concept, but the practical reality that grounds our hope.

All people, as well as all of creation, suffer. Suffering came into the world through sin—the sin of Adam and Eve in the Garden of Eden (Gen 3). It is perpetuated by the sin evident in society, its structures and ourselves. We all experience the effects of sin. The destructive forces of natural disasters, illness and injury do not discriminate between the just and the unjust (Mt 5:45).

Although some problems are the direct result of a person's sin—bitterness, pride, violence, sexual promiscuity, substance abuse, lifestyle choices—most suffering results from the general effects of evil in the world. We cannot blame an individual for his or her suffering. Suffering is simply part of life in a fallen world (1 Pet 4:12-19).

In the process, God uses suffering to teach and refine us. He lovingly walks with us through suffering (Is 43:1-7), assuring us that he will not allow anything more than we can bear (Heb 12:3-13). Our own suffering equips us to empathize with others in their suffering (Rom 5:1-5; 2 Cor 1:3-11). A nurse who has not suffered personally will find great difficulty providing emotional and spiritual support for others.

Nursing directly enters the suffering of this world, bringing the hope of comfort, strength and healing. Our taproot draws its nourishment from the words of Jesus, who instructed his followers: "Truly I tell you, just as you did it to one of the least of these who are members of my family, you did it to me" (Mt 25:40).

We actually proclaim the kingdom of God when we care for suffering people (Lk 4:18-21). Through Jesus Christ, God not only announced the ultimate end of suffering, he himself took human form to suffer for our sake—making that hope possible. Right now, we live in a now-and-not-yet kingdom. Jesus' suffering and death on the cross definitively won the victory over sin in our world. Our hope for a new world order is certain. But the effects of sin still ripple through our lives. The reality of the kingdom will not fully appear until the *parousia*—the second coming of Christ. In the meantime, we endure suffering with pa ience and hope, trusting in God's mercy and compassion, but also reacning out in love to care for others who are suffering. Ultimately, we look forward to a time when illness, tears and suffering will have been wiped away—when nurses won't be needed!

12

The Paradox
of Death

I KNOW I SHOULDN'T LET DEATH BOTHER ME BECAUSE I'M A Christian," a hospice nurse remarked, "but after seeing so many people die, I hate death! I've also become paranoid about every little symptom I see in myself or my family—I immediately assume that it is the beginning of a terminal illness. I live in constant fear of death."

Continuous exposure to death and dying brought this hospice nurse face to face with the nagging fears all of us harbor. Most of us can deny the inevitability of death most of the time. We can talk about the beauty of heaven and the hope of eternal life with objectivity and little emotional involvement. However, for those who experience the death of a loved one, the diagnosis of terminal illness or constant exposure to dying patients, the coping measure of denial quickly fades. It is hard to deny what is so ominously real.

Christians are not immune to death and grief. Like other people, they suffer from the agony of death because life has meaning, relationships have depth and importance, and we are strongly aware of all the unfinished business in this life. Few of us are as confident as the apostle Paul, who could say,

For to me, living is Christ and dying is gain. If I am to live in the flesh, that means fruitful labor for me; and I do not know which I prefer. I am hard pressed between the two: my desire is to depart and be with Christ, for that is far better; but to remain in the flesh is more necessary for you. (Phil 1:21-24)

Regardless of how much we love and trust God, most of us fear death. We do not want to be separated from our friends and family, even if it means moving on to a better life. Personally, I like this life. As much as I want to meet Jesus face to face, I'd much rather stay right here with my family in our comfortable, familiar home.

Avoiding the Subject

Because Christians often believe that fearing death shows lack of faith, the bereaved and dying among us may suffer neglect as well as grief. We either avoid them entirely because we do not know what to say, or we offer pious platitudes which further isolate them. For instance, a widow may have difficulty attending church services because she feels betrayed by Christian friends who never came to visit during the six months her husband lay dying of cancer. A mother who lost her daughter in an automobile accident six months ago is still wracked by grief, but her pastor tells her that she should be happy because her daughter is with the Lord. Now she feels guilty as well as depressed. Perhaps we show our lack of faith most clearly when we refuse to acknowledge the horror of death.

Even those Christians who have grappled with their own fear of death and believe they have overcome it find that it is a continuing struggle, not a one-time victory. Nurses who see death daily find themselves becoming gradually drained of life and hope. Roberta Paige, a hospice nurse, relates the following anecdote:

In a corner of the emergency department cubicle Ann sat with a chapel veil on her head praying the rosary. On the stretcher beside her lay Edward, her fiancé. Dark blood flowed through his nasogastric tube. He was also hemorrhaging from his rectum. Waxen and pale, Edward did not respond when I entered. He appeared to be asleep. Ann motioned me to her side and said that they were waiting for the Bishop to come, because Edward desperately wanted to be confirmed before he died.

The bishop came. Edward opened his eyes and smiled during the confirmation ritual. A short time later, he died.

The paradox of death seemed so evident in this place. The stench of blood and the sadness of a woman watching the man she loved ebb away countered the life that shined through Edward, more vividly perhaps because he was dying. As a Christian, I knew I should rejoice at this deathbed commitment to Christ. Instead, anger welled up inside me. I wanted to scream, "Death, I hate you!"[1]

Why does death threaten us so much? Why isn't the hope of eternal life with Christ sufficient to alleviate our fears? Doesn't the Bible say, "When this perishable body puts on imperishability, and this mortal body puts on immortality, then the saying that is written will be fulfilled: 'Death has been swallowed up in victory'" (1 Cor 15:54)? Perhaps we need to back up and look at what the Bible really does say about death.

The famous passage above from 1 Corinthians 15 is often quoted out of context. This sense of victory is not our present experience. The triumph is yet to come. We are not yet free from the sting of death. In the meantime, we are at war with an enemy. Earlier in the chapter we are told this:

> For as all die in Adam, so all will be made alive in Christ. But each in his own order: Christ the first fruits, then at his coming those who belong to Christ. Then comes the end, when he hands over the kingdom to God the Father, after he has destroyed every ruler and every authority and power. For he must reign until he has put all his enemies under his feet. The last enemy to be destroyed is death. (1 Cor 15:22-26)

We need not feel guilty about fearing death. Death is the ultimate enemy of God. It would be strange not to fear such an enemy.

Even Jesus struggled with death. He mourned at the tomb of his friend Lazarus, even though he knew he would raise him from the dead. John says he was "greatly disturbed in spirit and deeply moved" (Jn 11:33). The Greek terms imply a deep, agonized groaning. The death of a friend pained Jesus to the depths of his being.

Although Jesus went to his own death willingly, he did not go without extreme anguish. He wrestled in prayer, saying, "My Father, if it is possible, let this cup pass from me; yet not what I want but what you want" (Mt 26:39). Seeking support from his friends, he told his disciples, "I am deeply grieved, even to death; remain here, and stay awake with me" (Mt 26:38). Even Jesus needed comfort at the time of death.

The Inconvenience of Death

The disciples were not shining examples of supportive care. They fell asleep. Three times Jesus had to wake them and remind them of the seriousness of the situation and his need for them. But Jesus recognized their problem, saying, "The spirit indeed is willing, but the flesh is weak" (Mt 26:41). We can remember the disciples' weakness when our own care for dying patients falls short of the ideal. Jesus understands our failures too.

One incident in my (Judy's) experience continues to haunt me, reminding me that I would have done no better than the disciples in watching with Jesus. I was working three to eleven, the only R.N. on a hectic surgical unit with a reduced staff. Five patients returned from the recovery room on my shift. Nine others had intravenous drips and still needed frequent vital-sign checks. We had an emergency admission who needed extra attention. And in the room at the end of the hall was a woman in isolation, dying of hepatitis with her sixteen-year-old daughter at her side.

I didn't have time for a patient in isolation, or for a distraught teenager. The patient didn't belong on our floor anyway; she was a medical patient. She was hemorrhaging copiously from esophageal varices and aspirating blood despite a nasogastric tube. Her IV infiltrated. Her blood pressure was fading.

The daughter frantically began to shout, "Somebody do something!"

I paged the medical resident, who responded, "The woman is dying. Why should I come?"

In desperation I hustled the daughter out of the room and tried to clean up the patient and get her tubes in working order. As she left the room, the daughter told me, "If Mama's dying I want to be here!"

I closed the door and set to work, inwardly angry because I did not have time for this. As I removed the tape from the infiltrated IV catheter, the patient winced and said, "You don't have to be so mean." I felt a stab of guilt as I realized my anger was showing. Within minutes the woman died, her daughter waiting outside the door. Suddenly I felt consumed with guilt. Not only had I prevented the girl from spending those final moments with her mother, she was now alone with no one to comfort her. I had been "asleep" to the needs of the patient and her daughter because of my own inability to cope, just as Jesus' disciples slept while he suffered the agonies of death alone.

Death is almost always inconvenient. It defies our need for control and predictability. I could at least call the nursing supervisor to help me, but families whose lives are interrupted by the death of a loved one face a more drastic disruption. They may be left without a home or income. They may owe thousands of dollars in medical expenses. The loss of companionship and radical change in lifestyle may precipitate deep depression. Regardless of how carefully a family plans for death with wills, insurance policies, appointment of guardians and alternative housing, death is always a rude interruption. Even when death brings relief from pain and suffering, it is seldom easy for the survivors.

Terror and Hope

For the Christian, death is a paradox. It is both the hope of eternal life and the fear of the unknown. It is relief from pain and physical limitations—and the agony of separation. It is the joyous expectation of seeing God—and the fear of his wrath. It is universal (everyone must die), but each of us must die alone. It is the final release from all that binds us, and yet it is the ultimate enemy that came into the world through sin.

In the Scriptures death is both physical and spiritual. The greatest fear of the Old Testament writers was not physical death, but the anticipated separation from God. The psalmist cried out, "Is your steadfast love declared in the grave, or your faithfulness in Abaddon? Are your wonders known in the darkness, or your saving help in the land of forgetfulness?" (Ps 88:11-12).

The Old Testament writers believed that death meant a lack of relationship with God.[2] An understanding of this concept gives a fuller appreciation for the agony Jesus felt as he went to the cross, for his loss was total. His cry of "Eli, Eli, la'ma sabach-thani?" ("My God, my God, why have you forsaken me?") in Matthew 27:46 was his expression of terror at being separated from the Father even briefly. It is from that excruciating horror that we are freed by the death and resurrection of Jesus. But physical death remains, even for the Christian.

Herein we face another paradox. If the final victory over death is not yet realized, what happens to those who die in the interim? Jesus could tell the thief on the cross, "Today you will be with me in Paradise" (Lk 23:43), and Paul assures us that "neither death, nor life . . . nor anything else in all creation, will be able to separate us from the love of God in Christ Jesus our Lord" (Rom 8:38-39). But what happens between physical death and the second coming of Christ? One answer lies in 1 Thessalonians 4:13-18:

> But we do not want you to be uninformed, brothers and sisters, about those who have died, so that you may not grieve as others do who have no hope. For since we believe that Jesus died and rose again, even so, through Jesus, God will bring with him those who have died. For this we declare to you by the word of the Lord, that we who are alive, who are left until the coming of the Lord, will by no means precede those who have died. For the Lord himself, with a cry of command, with the archangel's call and with the sound of God's trumpet, will descend from heaven, and the dead in Christ will rise first. Then we who are alive, who are left, will be caught up in the clouds together with them to meet the Lord in the air; and so we will be with the Lord forever. Therefore encourage one another with these words.

Perhaps the key to understanding this passage lies in the Greek word *koimōmenōn*, which most Bible translations render as *sleeping*, but the NRSV translates as *died*. Sleep may be the closest experience we presently have for the concept of eternity. We go to sleep and awake with little or no sense of the time elapsed. The dead in Christ enter into eternity. They are freed from the constraints of time, so that "one day is as a thousand years, and a thousand years is as one day" (2 Pet 3:8). So Jesus could say to the thief on the cross, "*today* you will be with me in Paradise" (Lk 23:43). In eternity the kingdom of God has already come, because there is no time, but on earth we still await its coming.

Another paradox is that the Bible portrays death as both a natural event and an enemy. Genesis 25:8 reports, "Abraham breathed his last and died in a good old age, an old man and full of years, and was gathered to his people." Nothing could seem more natural and appropriate. Job 5:26 says, "You shall come to your grave in ripe old age, as a shock of grain comes up to the threshing floor in its season." Here death seems to almost fulfill the purpose for life.

Death presents us with a paradox of terror and hope. For many people the fear of God's judgment overshadows the hope of eternal life in Christ. Matthew 25:31-46 makes it clear that we will be judged for our actions (or inaction). Matthew 7:21 warns us that outward profession of faith is not sufficient for entrance into heaven. Jesus expects us to do "the will of my Father who is in heaven." The question of faith versus works can be confusing when reading such passages. According to James, though, works are the evidence of our faith (Jas 2:17). Those who truly belong to Christ will show the fruit of the Spirit in their attitudes and behavior (Gal 5:22-24). However, our salvation—our entrance into eternal life in Christ—is by grace alone. No record of good works is going to get us into heaven (Eph 2:8-9). Believers may endure discipline and even punishment from God for their own good (Heb 12:5-6), but they can rest assured of God's grace. Jesus assures us, "anyone who comes to me I will never drive away" (Jn 6:37).

Ending and New Beginning

Another biblical paradox about death is that it is both the end and a continuation of our life on earth. The relationship with God initiated on earth continues and grows in heaven. We also have the sure hope of being reunited with other believers after death. Looking to the future, death is merely a transition for the Christian. But looking backward, death is absolute and final. We cannot call back anyone from the dead. The Bible gives strong warnings that we are not to tamper with the realm of the dead (see, for example, Deut 18:10-12; Is 8:19; Luke 16:19-31).

Consulting the dead through seances, mediums, spirit guides, out-of-body experiences—or whatever the current fad may be—is off limits for Christians (Lev 19:31; Deut 18:9-14; Gal 5:19-21). In the first place, in doing so we merely deceive ourselves, for (except for Jesus and those he raised) the dead cannot return and communicate with us. But, more important, attempts to obtain hidden information from the dead show a blatant lack of faith in God. It is closely akin to Adam and Eve's act of disobedience in the garden of Eden where they were enticed by the serpent to gain forbidden knowledge so they could be "like God" (Gen 3). The Lord has revealed all that we need to know about death in order to live fully. We do not need to seek further insights from forbidden sources.

The paradox of death both frightens and intrigues us. It is perhaps at the thought of death that we are forced most clearly to consider the meaning of life. To a person who feels life has no meaning or purpose, death may seem a welcome release. On the other hand, a person with close relationships and a strong sense of purpose may hang onto life in the face of overwhelming obstacles.

Because death is universal, it is often called the "great equalizer." On the surface the statement appears to be true. Both rich and poor, famous and unknown, good and bad people die. The cliché "you can't take it with you" grew out of the realization that all of the things we accumulate on earth—wealth, possessions, power, status—are left behind at death. But for the Christian neither statement is entirely true, for we look beyond this earth to eternal life. There are a number of things we can take with us.

First of all, we take our relationship with God with us. In fact, Jesus is coming back to personally escort us into the presence of the Father (Jn 14:1-3). Although from this side of death we appear to die alone, in actuality the familiar words of the twenty-third psalm, "Even though I walk through the darkest valley, I fear no evil; for you are with me," tell us that this is merely a perception problem. We are not alone.

We can also take with us the expectation of reunion with Christians who have died before (and after) us (1 Thess 4:17). In eternity we will all be together; there will be no separation. We will have all the joys of human fellowship without the pain and suffering caused by sin in our earthly lives.

Finally, we can take our bodies with us. Not our aching, imperfect physical bodies, but "spiritual bodies," which will be recognizable, just as Jesus was when he returned from the grave (1 Cor 15:35-50). Death is not to become one with the universe or enter into a cycle of reincarnation. Neither is it the final stage of development. It is personally entering into the presence of the living God to worship and enjoy him forever (Rev 21:1-22:5).

Heaven and Hell

But what about those who die without Christ? As much as we would like to ignore this issue, judgment is the other side of the gospel message. There can be no "good news" until we first acknowledge the "bad news." John 3 tells us, "For God so loved the world that he gave his only Son, so that everyone who believes in him may not perish but may have eternal life" (v. 16). John goes on to explain, "Those who believe in him are not condemned; but those who do not believe are condemned already, because they have not believed in the name of the only Son of God" (v. 18).

The issue of judgment for the unbeliever puts the Christian nurse into a quandary. Nursing teaches us to be nonjudgmental, yet we cannot sit idly by and watch a dying unbeliever slip into eternal condemnation. Christian nurses vary in their responses. Some fly into a panic, becoming insensitive and obnoxious in their deathbed evangelism. Others say nothing but carry a growing burden of guilt over their failure to witness. Most of us fall somewhere in the middle of the spectrum of responses. Occasionally, we may experience the joy of leading someone to Christ. For the most part, we offer gentle physical and spiritual care, perhaps seeing a glimmer of faith sparked in our patients, but seldom see a deathbed conversion. Sometimes we feel guilty because we should have done more; other times we feel guilty because we were overbearing, straining the relationship with a patient.

Believer and unbeliever alike frequently ask the question, "How can a loving God send a person to hell?" There are no easy answers. Hell is a terrible end. Although the biblical picture of hell is varied and metaphorical, the one constant is that it is eternal separation from God (see, for example, Deut 32:22; Mt 5:22; 8:12; 10:28; 18:9; 22:13; 24:51; 25:30, 41; Lk 16:24; 2 Pet 2:4). We know from the Scriptures that God does not want anyone to go to hell (2 Pet 3:9). The whole purpose of Jesus Christ's birth, death and resurrection was to save us from eternal condemnation (Jn 3:16-17, 1 Tim 1:15). It is only those who choose to live apart from God who are condemned to hell (Jn 12:47-50), but at the point of death that choice becomes final and awful (Lk 13:23-30).

Stephen Travis puts the biblical concepts of heaven and hell into focus by defining them in the context of our relationship with God. "If this be so, we can see that both heaven and hell are best thought of not as a reward or punishment for the kind of life we have lived, but as the logical outcome of our relationship with God in this life. Heaven is not a reward for loving God any more than marriage is a reward for being engaged. And hell is not a punishment for turning one's back on Christ and choosing the road to destruction. It is where the road goes."[3]

Jesus gently but firmly bids us enter into a relationship with him that leads to eternal life. He calls us to recognize our own sinfulness—our natural inclination to put other things in a higher priority than knowing and loving God. He brings us to a sense of our humanity—realizing that we are not ultimately in power and control. He then reveals to us that he has assumed full responsibility for our sin. When we respond in repentance, belief and obedience to him, he enters into our lives and begins a lifelong process of changing us to be like him.

God does not force us into relationship with himself. Jesus did not run after the rich young man who approached him in Matthew 11:22. He let the man go away sorrowful when his possessions held higher value for him than eternal life. Jesus faithfully proclaimed the gospel, but there is no record of his using high-pressure tactics with anyone. His example suggests that we can relax in our approach to dying patients. If a person refuses to discuss spiritual things or actively denies God, we must respect that choice. If we have been faithful in ministering God's love through word and deed, we need not feel guilty about a person's eternal destiny.

Perhaps the most honest position to take on the fate of unbelievers is to admit that we cannot know for certain. The Bible does not tell us exactly what will happen to those who have never heard the gospel, or the mentally handicapped, or babies or young children. When a person's commitment to Christ seems questionable, we need not necessarily despair. Only God knows the true spiritual state of a person. All that we know for certain is that God gives us the opportunity to respond in faith now, and he invites us to join him in spreading the joyful news of his love and mercy. It is not our place to assign people to heaven or hell. Our job is to proclaim and be faithful (Jas 4:17). What we do know for certain is that God loves each person far more than we ever could, and that he is just. We can trust those in our care to him.

Yes, death for the Christian is still an enemy. It separates us from our loved ones. Death disrupts normal family functioning. It can be exorbitantly expensive, especially when preceded by a long illness. The process of dying can be ugly and painful. Death is filled with unknowns. But for the Christian there is hope in death.

The hope of eternal life is the knowledge that our relationship with Jesus Christ will remain unbroken in death. We have sampled the goodness of God here on earth. We look forward to basking in the pure, full presence of God after death, no longer afflicted by physical suffering, emotional struggles or broken relationships. All that is true, honorable, just, lovely, gracious, excellent and praiseworthy (Phil 4:8) will surround us. We will know the love of God in ways in which human love has never reached us. We cannot even imagine the depths of its goodness.

Think about what it would be like to go to a party with all the people you ever wanted to see, and to be able to have a mutually caring relationship with each one. Imagine experiencing the pure love and joy of being with your parents and siblings without any of the old dysfunctional patterns. Consider the deep friendships that somehow dissolved in pain and misunderstanding suddenly being restored to their original luster. In heaven, no longer will we know loneliness, fear, anger or frustration. We will be able to love and be loved as God loves us. What a party!

Practical Considerations

In the meantime the church has been commissioned to be a small taste of heaven. When the church functions as God intends, it offers mutual love and support throughout life, and especially in times of crisis. We uphold one another in prayer as well as providing practical assistance. At the time of death, that may include offering food, transportation, housing, money and companionship for the family. The funeral service serves to reassure the bereaved of the hope of eternal life and provides concrete human comfort and support.

Dr. Paul Johnson, a physician who faced a life-threatening illness, suggests the following guidelines for Christians when supporting a dying person:

□ Always tell the truth.

□ Never set times.

□ Listen with sensitivity.

□ Respond to needs.

□ Never allow the person to feel abandoned.

□ Make yourself available.

□ Don't give medical advice.

□ If necessary protect persons from themselves (especially if they are self-medicating or not following their prescribed medical regimen).

□ Always hold out hope.

□ Provide spiritual support.[4]

Johnson describes his own feelings as he battled cancer.

> Partly it was embarrassment. All of a sudden I was different: someone somehow inferior, abnormal. Then, too, just as suddenly, I was the focus of attention, but it was a strange kind of attention. Not really personal, but impersonal, as I was the object of tests and examinations and all sorts of sterile routines. All of this seemed aimed at making me pull back, within myself, away from relationships which were now impersonal and professional rather than personal and caring.[5]

In this time of extreme isolation and loneliness, Donley's three nursing approaches in suffering will provide comfort and hope.

First, we can offer compassionate accompaniment. We can listen carefully to the sick or dying person's needs and concerns, pray with the person and share appropriate Scripture passages. We can work to facilitate reconciliation in broken relationships. Sometimes we may need to merely stay with the person and say nothing.

Second, we can help to bring meaning into the situation and to the person's life. Encouraging reminiscence, family sharing and worship will focus the person's attention on what is most important in their life. Recalling favorite hymns, Bible passages and family stories help to put a person's life into a larger context.

Finally, we can provide excellent physical care. Pain control and other comfort measures, as well as a pleasant environment, make it easier for a dying person to relax and to relate to loved ones. Gentle, loving touch is particularly important at this point. A backrub, a hand on the shoulder, or holding a person's hand, communicates human warmth and care. Not only should we consciously work toward caring touch in our own interactions with the dying person, but we may also need to encourage family members and friends to touch. They may hesitate to do so for fear of hurting the person, or they may feel intimidated by the hospital environment and medical equipment.

Nurses in churches have a particularly important role in educating the Christian community in how to care for dying people and their families. Family members may feel trapped and isolated if they are caring for someone at home. They may also need help to know how to provide the physical care the dying person requires. Simple things like giving a bedbath, making an occupied bed, lifting, transferring and assisting the person with eating and toiletting may feel overwhelming to a family member who has never done them before. We can offer instruction and support to them, as well as arranging volunteer help when needed. A nurse's assessment skills can be invaluable for a church congregation in knowing how to handle such situations.

Hospice nurses often provide an outstanding service to dying patients and their families. They manage pain, facilitate communication with the family and health care personnel, provide emotional and spiritual support, arrange for practical concerns such as transportation, housekeeping and meal preparation and offer follow-up care for the family. When a person is dying at home, the hospice nurses remain on call to assist the family, preparing them to know what to do at the time of death and supporting them in the process.

In the case of a sudden death, family members will not have the benefit of hospice care or any preparation for the sudden onslaught of emotions and tasks to be done. Our role, unless we are working within a congregational setting, will be brief and limited. The most important intervention we can make at this point is to connect the family with their faith community by calling their pastor or the hospital chaplain. Nurses in churches will be especially important in helping these families deal with grief and face the complex decisions they will have to make in the coming months.

Nurses in churches can also provide or arrange for instruction in the practical planning and decision-making that need to take place surrounding death. Many congregations encourage their people to pre-plan funerals and keep their desires on file in the church office. Churches with senior citizen groups or parish nurses may sponsor classes on how to handle Medicare, develop advanced directives and wills, or choose an extended-care facility. Many hospices will send a speaker to church groups to explain their services. Churches may also sponsor grief support groups. If your own congregation does not offer these services, you can develop a list of community resources, including other churches, to which you can refer people.

The church and the individual members within it are in the business of life and living. For that reason, Christian fellowship is essential for the person who works with death and dying on a daily basis. Family caregivers need to attend worship and other church functions. Hospice volunteers or trained church members may be able to relieve them so they can get away. Nurses also need the support of the church. The constant exposure to death which nurses in oncology, hospice and critical care face can become over-whelmingly depressing. Bible study, prayer, worship and mutual support and encouragement reaffirm the hope to which we are called—a hope that leads to life, not death.

Death is the last enemy. Even for Christians, death painfully interrupts and reorders our lives. However, though we grieve, it is not "as others do who have no hope" (1 Thess 4:13). We do not grieve alone. The Christian community surrounds and upholds us. We do not die alone. Jesus assured us, "Do not let your hearts be troubled. Believe in God, believe also in me. In my Father's house there are many dwelling places. If it were not so, would I have told you that I go to prepare a place for you? And if I go and prepare a place for you, I will come again and will take you to myself, so that where I am, there you may be also" (Jn 14:1-3).

In the face of death Jesus offers us hope of eternal life. As Christian nurses, we offer that hope to those who walk through the valley of the shadow of death.

Part Five

Nursing as a Response of Faith

13

Nursing as
Christian Caring

T HE FIRST TWELVE CHAPTERS OF THIS BOOK HAVE EXAMINED the concepts in the nursing metaparadigm from a Christian perspective. Now the task remains to define nursing today. Who are we? What do we do? While the definition of nursing has gradually evolved over time, in recent years there has been a radical shift in perspective.

We have seen how nursing as a public role first developed in the Christian church but by the seventeenth century had degenerated into a sorry state. When Pennsylvania Hospital, the first hospital in America, opened in 1752, nursing care was provided by both male and female nurses who were expected to be "trustworthy and experienced" but had no formal training. Their duties, which included preparing food and feeding patients, washing and ironing the linens and keeping the rooms clean, were shared by the patients as they were able.[1] However, during this period nursing occurred primarily within the family as an extension of motherhood. Hospital nursing was not considered a respectable vocation for a young woman.

Emily Hitchens and Lilyan Snow contend that volunteer nurses during the American Civil War "invented nursing" out of necessity. They volunteered because they felt it was the right thing to do, because the wounds of battle required care. The care these nurses offered included "order, cleanliness, and food when it was possible, and simple *being with* at all times." Many of these nurses went on to establish schools of nursing after the war.[2]

As we have seen, the Crimean War forced Florence Nightingale to reinvent nursing. She defined nursing as having "charge of the personal health of somebody . . . [knowing] how to put the constitution in such a state as it will have no disease, or that it will recover from disease."[3] She believed that every woman was a nurse and wrote her little book, *Notes on Nursing*, to help them "think how to nurse."[4] The women she took with her to Scutari were not formally educated as nurses. Nightingale taught them after they arrived. Following the war she established the first secular school of nursing.

However, war alone did not define nursing. Catholic monastic orders maintained the role of nursing sisters throughout the history of the church. The nineteenth century brought a revival of nursing in the Protestant church, especially in northern Europe. The deaconess movement sprang up as a response to the gospel. These early deaconesses lived in community and cared for the sick and poor without charge. They established hospitals and schools of nursing, training many women (including Florence Nightingale).[5]

The nuns and deaconesses were never overly concerned about defining nursing; they just did it. When the nuns first arrived in America in the eighteenth century, they weren't trained as nurses but as teachers. But they found that the people they had come to teach needed health care, so they started a hospital and nursed. Others became social workers, but when health needs surfaced, they too became nurses.[6] The deaconesses demonstrated a similar flexibility. Their primary commitment was not to a professional discipline, but to God and service.[7] This strength may have led to the eventual decline of Christian nursing. The pursuit of a "secular order" by Nightingale and the early public health nurses in America meant that nurses caught the optimistic spirit of the age more quickly than the call to Christian commitment.

In the early part of the twentieth century, secular nursing was still not clearly defined, but to a large extent nurses became physicians' assistants, a role that still shapes the public image of nursing. In an attempt to provide nursing with a stronger identity, set standards for nursing education and work toward greater autonomy, nurses began to organize into state and national associations. A body of thoughtful literature began to develop as a growing number of professional nursing journals began publication. These associations and journals became a forum for discussing the nature of nursing. World War II set the stage for increasing activism and assertiveness among nurses, and by 1946 the American Nurses Association had a plan for the future that included improved working conditions, educational standards with federal subsidies and increased professional organization.[8]

In 1955 the American Nurses Association approved a definition of nursing practice that was adopted by most state boards of nursing:

> The practice of professional nursing means the performance for compensation of any act in the observation, care, and counsel of the ill, injured, or infirm, or the maintenance of health or prevention of illness of others, or in the supervision and teaching of other personnel, or the administration of medications and treatment as prescribed by a licensed physician or dentist; requiring substantial specialized judgment and skill and based on knowledge and application of the principles of biological, physical, and social science. The foregoing shall not be deemed to include acts of diagnosis or prescription of therapeutic or corrective measures.[9]

This definition made a clear break with the tradition of volunteer nursing or Christian communities providing care without charge. Professional nursing required compensation. This focus on compensation would become a rising theme. Another significant contrast to the nursing of nuns and deaconesses also occurred. While the nurse's responsibilities of observing, caring, counseling, supervising and teaching seem to be a step toward autonomy, the definition engraved the physicians' assistant role into nurse practice acts. Nurses were not allowed to diagnose or treat. Treatments and medications could be prescribed only by a physician.

While the ANA definition remained the legal definition of nursing, the 1950s and 1960s brought a ferment of thinking about the nature of nursing.

New definitions began to emerge. They focused more on nursing's unique-ness and less on its subservience to medicine. Virginia Henderson's classic definition of nursing, discussed in chapter one, has been ingrained into nurses ever since it was adopted in 1960. Most nurses feel this definition in their gut. It identifies who we are, what we are concerned about and what we do. It also allows for an increasing sense of autonomy.

All of these early definitions focus on maintaining and restoring health to the individual and assume a positive direction toward health (or peaceful death). But by 1980 new definitions began to proliferate. Some of them were based on radically different understandings of nursing concepts. The American Nurses Association's 1980 *Nursing: A Social Policy Statement* definition did not even articulate the promotion of human health as the goal of nursing care.[11] The statement defined nursing as the "diagnosis and treatment of human responses to actual and potential health problems."[12] It was an attempt to get around the prohibitions against diagnosing and treating disease in nurse practice acts.

In response to protests about the lack of focus in the 1980 definition, the 1995 revision of this statement maintains the original wording, but adds that more recent definitions "frequently acknowledge four essential features of contemporary nursing practice":

☐ attention to the full range of human experiences and responses to health and illness without restriction to a problem-focused orientation

☐ integration of objective data with knowledge gained from an under-standing of the patient or group's subjective experience

☐ application of scientific knowledge to the processes of diagnosis and treatment

☐ provision of a caring relationship that facilitates health and healing[13]

This revision also states that "nurses intervene to promote health, prevent illness, or assist with activities that contribute to recovery from illness or to achieving a peaceful death."[14] Although this definition seems more in line with Florence Nightingale's, nursing is no longer the calling of every woman. It is a "scientific discipline as well as a profession"[15] that requires education (with a baccalaureate degree recommended) and national exami-nation for licensure. Furthermore, this definition takes a bolder step toward the issue of diagnosing and treating. However, its scope of practice remains fuzzy, with a "flexible boundary that is responsive to the changing needs of society and the expanding knowledge base of its theoretical and scientific domains."[16]

Nurse practice acts in most states now permit advanced practice nurses to make simple diagnoses and prescribe certain classes of drugs, further blurring the line between nursing and medicine.[17] Nurses can practice independently, own and manage extended care facilities, establish their own companies to deliver care and receive compensation from third party payers. Insurance companies now hire nurses as case managers with the authority to grant or deny reimbursements for physician-ordered medications and treatments.

Nursing's frantic scrambling to redefine itself in order to advance (or even survive), together with the current upheaval in health care delivery, presents us with an opportunity to reassess where we have come in nursing and determine where we want to go. To do so, we need to back up and look at nursing through a Christian worldview. Reacting from the midst of the whirlwind and jumping on the current trends without thoughtful examination could prove disastrous for nursing. Many of today's trends are contradictory and lead to fragmentation of the profession. There is tremendous growth in the move toward more education (nursing master's degrees and doctorates), while in other sectors the trend is toward less education (institutional training and associate degrees). Nurses are gaining more autonomy (advanced practice, community health, entrepreneurship) but becoming more isolated and alienated from one another in the process. Parish nursing brings nursing back into the church, but it often finds its funding through health care conglomerates, which then control its continuing education and supervision.

In the midst of all this defining and redefining, just what is *Christian* nursing? How do we gain the perspective needed to define it? Many contemporary nursing leaders (and theologians) are saying that we are defined by our stories. To some degree, that works. Throughout nursing history we can catch a glimpse of what Patricia Donahue calls the *nursing impulse,* a uniting of "the head, the heart and the hands" to nurture health and overcome disease.[18] However, there are also low points and digressions in the story of nursing that we do not want to incorporate into our identity. Rather, we need to repent of our self-interest and neglect and turn again to Jesus Christ for our vision of nursing.

Instead of looking primarily to nursing history or even current practice to find our story, we must begin with God's story in the Scriptures, for that is where Christian nursing began. The term *nurse* in the Bible implied a woman who fed and cared for infants and young children, not today's professional role. However, health care figured prominently in the life and teachings of Jesus. He healed the sick, cared for the poor and oppressed, sought out those whom society rejected, and instructed his followers to go and do likewise. Health care—including the physical, psychosocial and spiritual dimensions—soon became the concern of the whole church.

Several characteristics of Christian nursing stand out in the Scriptures. (1) Nursing is a response to God's grace that flows from a dynamic personal relationship with God. (2) It is a ministry of the church and functions in the context of the body of Christ. (3) It recognizes the role of sin in a world created good, and it seeks to restore justice and righteousness. (4) It views the person as created in the image of God. (5) It works toward the goal of *shalom* as ultimate health. (6) It is demonstrated in compassionate care that is characterized by the fruit of the Spirit. These characteristics, and the theological understanding of the concepts in the nursing paradigm presented in the first twelve chapters, will help us both to define nursing and to shape the future of nursing practice.

Based on these considerations, we will define Christian nursing as *a ministry of compassionate care for the whole person, in response to God's grace toward a sinful world, which aims to foster optimum health* (shalom) *and bring comfort in suffering and death for anyone in need.*

A Ministry

Ministry in the New Testament and the early church was understood to be the work of every Christian. The Greek term translated as ministry, *diakonia,* essentially means service. It incorporates everything from preaching the gospel to waiting on tables and delivering relief to the poor. Jesus demonstrated this spirit of service by washing his disciples' feet, then telling them to follow his example (Jn 13). In fact, the term *diakonos* (servant) is often used synonymously with *doulos* (slave). When Jesus' disciples began to seek power and privilege, he told them: "But it is not so among you; but whoever wishes to become great among you must be your servant, and whoever wishes to be first among you must be slave of all" (Mk 10:43-44).

The ministry of nursing is servant work. Sometimes it is dirty work like washing feet and emptying bedpans. It is the visiting nurse who returns on her day off to clean a patient's apartment, or buys dressings for a patient who can't afford them. It is the critical-care nurse who works double shifts to cover for a sick colleague. It is the nurse practitioner who gives up a lucrative position to work in an inner-city clinic that pays less than he made before his advanced-practice certification. It is the nursing instructor who spends extra hours encouraging and counseling students. It is the nursing leader who pours tremendous time and energy into serving on a professional organization's task force to develop documents that will shape the future of nursing. It is the nurse who gets involved in the political system to work for justice in health delivery.

To a large extent these servant-nurses remain unheralded and invisible.[19] But the key to servanthood comes in whom we are serving. Jesus said, "Truly I tell you, just as you did it to one of the least of these who are members of my family, you did it to me" (Mt 25:40). We are servants of the Lord Jesus Christ, who also said to us, "I do not call you servants any longer, because the servant does not know what the master is doing; but I have called you friends, because I have made known to you everything that I have heard from my Father" (Jn 15:15).

Within the body of Christ, each person is equipped with various gifts for ministry. Romans 12:6-8 lists ministry *(diakonia)* among other gifts: "We have gifts that differ according to the grace given to us: prophecy, in proportion to faith; ministry, in ministering; the teacher, in teaching; the exhorter, in exhortation; the giver, in generosity; the leader, in diligence; the compassionate, in cheerfulness." In this passage "ministering" more likely referred to nursing than to anything resembling the ordained pastorate (which did not exist in this period). The gifts are not mutually exclusive.

Those who minister may also have gifts of prophecy, teaching, exhortation, generosity, leadership or compassion. Paul simply instructs us to use the gifts God has given.

First Corinthians 12:4-12 provides a more extensive explanation of spiritual gifts.

> Now there are varieties of gifts, but the same Spirit; and there are varieties of services, but the same Lord; and there are varieties of activities, but it is the same God who activates all of them in everyone. To each is given the manifestation of the Spirit for the common good. To one is given through the Spirit the utterance of wisdom, and to another the utterance of knowledge according to the same Spirit, to another faith by the same Spirit, to another gifts of healing by the one Spirit, to another the working of miracles, to another prophecy, to another the discernment of spirits, to another various kinds of tongues, to another the interpretation of tongues. All these are activated by one and the same Spirit, who allots to each one individually just as the Spirit chooses.
>
> For just as the body is one and has many members, and all the members of the body, though many, are one body, so it is with Christ.

Notice that the gifts are intended to fit together for the benefit of the whole body. Today when nurses are clamoring for autonomy, we have to recognize that Christian nursing is never an autonomous role. The Christian nurse functions as part of the body of Christ and is always accountable to the church (even when in secular employment). Because health care is the concern of the whole church, the boundaries of nursing's ministry will always remain fuzzy.

The history of nursing and compassionate health care is intricately woven through church history—until fairly recently. It was when nursing moved away from its association with the church that it degenerated into an independent profit-making scheme practiced by the Sairey Gamps of Dickens's day. We are seeing a similar decline today as hospitals and health care agencies, which were once church-owned and operated, have become dependent on federal funds and then on conglomerate buyouts for survival.

If nursing is a part of the body of Christ that has been particularly gifted with the ability and responsibility to care for the health needs of others, then one of our primary roles must be to awaken the church to its mission of healing. Jesus sent out his followers in Luke 10:8-9, saying: "Whenever you enter a town and its people welcome you . . . cure the sick who are there, and say to them, 'The kingdom of God has come near to you.' " Proclamation is only half of Jesus' commission. Demonstration of the gospel through compassionate health care is the other half.

Compassionate Care

Jesus gave the most comprehensive description of compassionate care when he told the story of the good Samaritan in Luke 10:30-35:

> A man was going down from Jerusalem to Jericho, and fell into the hands of robbers, who stripped him, beat him, and went away, leaving him half dead. . . . But a Samaritan while traveling came near him; and when he saw him, he was moved with pity. He went to him and bandaged his wounds, having poured oil and wine on them. Then he put him on his own animal, brought him to an inn, and took care of him. The next day he took out two denarii, gave them to the innkeeper, and said, "Take care of him; and when I come back, I will repay you whatever more you spend."

The Samaritan in this story had no legal responsibility to stop and help. Two Jewish religious leaders had already passed by the wounded man without getting involved. The victim was presumably a Jewish man, and customarily Jews were the enemies of Samaritans. The man could have been a decoy set up by the robbers in order to claim another victim. Yet the Samaritan pitied the man and risked his own welfare to intervene, using his own limited supplies. Furthermore, he took his patient to an inn and stayed with him as long as he could, then provided for continuity of care after he left.

Although caring has always been central to nursing, there is little consensus about what caring means. One group of researchers identified twenty-three different definitions of caring in the nursing literature (and they missed a few). They divided these definitions into five major categories: caring as (1) a human trait, (2) a moral imperative, (3) an affect, (4) an interpersonal interaction and (5) a therapeutic intervention.[20] Only the last one (under which only six definitions fit) involves any kind of physical care. How do these definitions compare with a Christian view of caring?

We do not need to look far to realize that caring for others is not intrinsic to human nature. Empirical evidence surrounds us attesting to the opposite; so does the biblical witness. Romans 3:23 tells us that "all have sinned and fall short of the glory of God." The good Samaritan was remarkable because his compassionate care stood in contrast to the normal human response (illustrated by the two religious leaders who did not stop to help). During a recent class for CPR recertification, the instructor told us, "Outside of a health care setting no one has to know that you are a nurse or that you are certified in CPR—the risks are just too great to get involved." Most of the class nodded in agreement. Caring for strangers is not intrinsic to human nature. Even within the health care setting, there seems to be a common human bent toward leaving the dirty work for the next shift.

On the other hand, the second category of definitions—caring as a moral imperative—may well develop in a culture shaped by strong moral virtues. Such was the case of the "nursing inventors" in the nineteenth century, who were influenced by the philosophy of Immanuel Kant. They sought to retain Christianity's values without the religious commitment, making it into a practical morality. However, caring as a moral imperative does not develop in a vacuum (or in a pluralistic society). It is not a general principle that seems obvious to every reasonable person. It develops in the context of a living relationship with Jesus Christ within the body of Christ, which informs the standards for the virtue of love (which in turn results in caring). Once the spiritual foundations fade from memory, the virtues begin to crumble. While the good Samaritan demonstrated caring, it was not out of any categorical imperative. He was simply "moved with pity."

Whose values set the moral standards for caring in today's nursing? In Eastern philosophy caring happens primarily in the mind, through seeking enlightenment. For the naturalist, caring usually means doing what is "best" for society rather than the individual. To many postmodernists morality is simply what seems good to an individual at the time. Without a common religious foundation, we lose our categories for categorical imperatives. When a person can pick and choose the basis for caring by personal preference, previously unethical behavior such as partial-birth abortions and physician-assisted (and nurse-assisted) suicide can be touted by their supporters as caring practices, or health maintenance organizations can justify huge profits at the expense of adequate coverage.

The third category, caring as an affect or emotion, is not very helpful in the real world of nursing. We are all faced with patients we just don't like. In fact, our first response to some patients may well be revulsion—but we still must care for them. When the Good Samaritan cared for the wounded man beside the road, although he was moved with pity, he probably felt no great love for him. In fact, this patient was so repulsive that others crossed to the other side of the road instead of caring for him. The Samaritan's compassion was demonstrated instead by concrete physical acts of mercy—by touching the patient, cleaning his wounds and staying with him while he recovered.

The fourth category, caring as an interpersonal interaction, depends on meaningful, respectful communication between the nurse and the patient. That works only if the patient is alert and cooperative. The wounded man in the good Samaritan story was left "half dead." I doubt that any meaningful interaction occurred. He was probably unconscious. We need to care for people even when they are unable to articulate their needs or care for us in return. Most nursing care is a one-way deal. We can delight in those rare encounters when we feel cared for in return by a patient, but we can't base our model of caring on reciprocal need-meeting.

Nursing theorists using a New Paradigm worldview often assume that caring comes naturally to nurses and that it occurs as a metaphysical event. It usually means just "being with" a person. Compassionate accompaniment is an important element in our nursing care—but we cannot stop there. Psychiatric nurse Verna Carson expresses concern about this view because "defining our caring role as 'being with' . . . seems to exclude the very important aspects of 'doing for' and 'doing with.' "[21] Dunlop also notes that the emerging concept of caring in nursing seems to "ignore the body and its associated physical care."[22] But this is not the understanding of caring we see in the Scriptures. What would have happened if the Good Samaritan had simply sat down at the side of the road with the wounded man without making any active interventions? Both would probably have been killed by robbers or wild animals.

Caring in the Bible

The Bible gives us a very clear picture of what caring means, and it is essentially a therapeutic intervention. We learn about caring by looking at God. "Cast all your anxiety on him [God], because he cares for you" (1 Pet 5:7). How does God care for us? A brief biblical overview paints a vivid and comforting picture.

We begin in Genesis 1 where God creates a man and a woman, declares them *good* and enters into relationship with them. By Genesis 3, the man and woman have tested the limits and disobeyed God, bringing upon themselves all the ugly effects of sin—pain, suffering and death. But already at this awful moment we begin to see God's care demonstrated. He makes clothes for them (Gen 3:21). Then the long history of God gently meeting his people's needs unfolds.

God's involvement in the lives of his people is practical and physical. In Hosea 11, we see God's care expressed in his calling Israel, teaching him to walk, holding him in his arms, healing him, easing his work load and bending down to feed him. Jeremiah tells us that God restores health and heals wounds (30:17). Zechariah says that God cares for his flock by changing unjust systems (10:3). These themes are repeated in Matthew 6:25-31, where Jesus tells us that our lives and bodies are important to God and that he will provide food, clothing and shelter to sustain us.

We see an interesting twist to the "just being with" understanding of care in Isaiah 43:1-3. Here God says that he created and formed us, called us by name, claims us as his own, then walks with us *to protect us* when we go through the tough experiences of life. This is no mere presence—it is a sacrificial involvement in our lives. That sacrifice culminates in God's being willing to give his Son to die for us in the crucifixion of Jesus.

Christian caring is not just an emotional tug, an intellectual concept or a metaphysical event. It is hands-on, patient-centered, physical, psychoso-cial and spiritual intervention to meet the needs of a patient *regardless of how the nurse feels*. In the process of nursing we may eventually develop a caring affect, but our ability to feel caring will continue to be challenged by the system and by obnoxious patients.

Our skill in caring develops as we receive care from others and, ultimately, as we grow in our understanding and acceptance of God's care for us. Caring is an act of faith, for it involves the risk of opening ourselves to another who may not want to care or be cared for. But unless we take that risk we cannot claim to be truly nursing.

Nursing doesn't hold an exclusive claim to caring. Lots of people care—parents, friends, social workers, pastors, teachers. Paul told the Thessaloni-ans, "We were gentle among you, like a nurse taking care of her children" (1 Thess 2:7). But nursing means providing compassionate care for the whole person, in response to God's grace toward a sinful world, which aims to foster optimum health and bring comfort in suffering for anyone in need. It means getting our hands (and often our clothing) dirty and putting ourselves at risk for the welfare of our patients. A body of knowledge, an attitude of service and a vital relationship with God are required to make that caring truly Christian nursing.

For the Whole Person

Christian nursing is holistic, caring for the person physically, emotionally, psychosocially and spiritually. In fact, we know that ultimate healing cannot occur unless our patients are placed in the hands of Jesus, the Great Physician (Is 53:5). However, a nurse's background in the physical and social sciences, as well as the nursing arts, provides unique qualifications to care for the physical needs of others and to understand human responses to illness. Nursing, because of its concern for the whole person, is also uniquely positioned to coordinate communications among members of an interdis-ciplinary health care team.

A pastor recently told us about a pastoral call he made accompanied by Sue, a nurse from his congregation. He expressed amazement over how much more information Sue uncovered in one visit than he had gained in over a year. By simply observing the woman and her surroundings and initiating a brief conversation, Sue assessed that she had some potentially serious health problems and that she needed help with her diet, transportation, laundry and housekeeping. Sue was then able to help her receive the services she needed from community agencies and volunteers in the church.

This pastor's story is one we have heard over and over. Nurses just have a different way of seeing, hearing, smelling, feeling and perceiving—a skill that develops over years of experience. Perhaps that is one of our primary spiritual gifts. A comment made by a nurse visiting an extended-care facility illustrates this kind of perception. She stopped, looked around and remarked, "This is a good nursing home. It smells good, and there is a light in the residents' eyes." Two very simple observations, but they indicated that residents were receiving good physical care and also respect and loving attention.

We examined in chapter seven what it means to be human, but let's summarize the main points again. First, all people are created by God in his image (Gen 1:26) to live in loving relationship with God, self and others (Deut 6:4-6; Mt 22:37-39) and as responsible stewards of the environment (Gen 1:26). Second, every person is separated from God by sin, but that relationship is restored by grace through faith in Jesus Christ, in whom we are redeemed and made holy by the Holy Spirit (Rom 3:22-28; 1 Cor 6:11). Third, the person is a physically, psychosocially and spiritually integrated being with intrinsic value and significance (Ps 8:4-8; 1 Thess 5:23; Heb 2:11-17). Fourth, each person is responsible to live a healthful lifestyle (1 Cor 3:16-17; Eph 5:29) and to promote health (Ex 15:26; 3 Jn 2), but also to find meaning in suffering and death (Rom 5:3-5; 1 Cor 15:54; 1 Thess 4:13-14).

Nurses care for all dimensions of the person as they relate to health and healing. If any of these aspects of the person is ignored, healing will usually be impeded. Therefore, nursing assessment must include not only biological functioning but social, emotional and spiritual factors as well.

A Response to God's Grace Toward a Sinful World
The motivation for Christian nursing comes primarily from a sense of

gratitude to God, not merely a reaction to human need or a sense of duty (although they too flow naturally from a grateful heart). We can say with the apostle John, "We love, because he [God] first loved us" (1 Jn 4:19). The contrast between gratitude and duty results primarily in a difference in attitude and approach. When I care out of a sense of gratitude for what God has done for me, I can view the patient as a person of great value, worthy of my respect, interest and attention. When I care out of a sense of duty, the patient becomes an object. I do what I have to do and get out. The spirit of that fine line is expressed in a letter written by a nurse in an extended-care facility—written to one of the patients, after he died.

> Your reputation preceded my meeting you, Robert. My coworkers called you "Starman"—they said they believed you were communicating with the stars. I found out what they meant. When I worked third shift and checked on you throughout the night, your eyes were always open, as though gazing into lost galaxies of time.
>
> Frankly, sometimes we felt repulsed by your twisted figure. Forgive our shallow thinking. Anyhow, thanks for allowing me to bathe you, to feed you and care for you.
>
> I cannot imagine having to be cared for through so many years, dependent on someone for all your life-sustaining needs. I pray that every hand that touched you touched with compassion, and every word spoken was with loving kindness. But I know as I write this, that was not the case. God forgive us.[23]

Even as we care out of a sense of gratitude, there is always a sense that God is still working on us, making us more like Christ (2 Cor 3:18). We don't always care in the way we would like to care. Sometimes only a sense of duty enables us to press on. We humbly struggle with our own sinfulness, our inability to truly care and to draw our strength from him (Phil 4:13).

Aims to Foster Optimum Health

Health is being able to live as God created us to be—as an integrated whole, living in loving relationship with God, self and others (Ps 16). Health cannot be separated into isolated compartments, and neither can nursing care. We deceive ourselves when we think that we can care only for physical needs while ignoring the emotional, spiritual and social needs of our patients. If we are concerned only for the mechanical functioning of the body, we would do better as pure scientists or car mechanics. On the other hand, we cannot fully meet the health needs of anyone while ignoring physical needs. Pastors and counselors focus on the spiritual and emotional components of health, but only nurses incorporate all dimensions. We need not duplicate the services of other members of the health care team, but we often function as coordinators of care, making referrals, communicating across the disciplines and keeping the whole person in view.

The presence of sin in the world and the predilection of each person to sin take a toll on health spiritually, physically and psychosocially (Ex 20:5; Ps 32:3-4; Lk 5:17-25). Physical or psychosocial dysfunction can cause spiritual distress (Job 16:7-9; Ps 13—22). Nurses stand in a unique position to assess the interrelationship between these dimensions.

The intimacy required in caring for the body often leads patients to be more open in sharing emotional and spiritual concerns. For example, a woman who feels guilt over a past abortion may feel freer to confess her sense of guilt to the nurse, who already knows her medical history, than to a pastor whom she perceives as "too holy" to understand. A man with bleeding ulcers may be able to tell a nurse about his anger toward his son or his alcohol binges but hesitate to seek professional counseling.

Nursing works toward the healing of the whole person in the context of communities. This broad understanding of health—*shalom*—is the goal of nursing. Furthermore, it is the goal of the entire Christian community and a sign of the kingdom of God (Rev 21:1-7). Within that broader view of health, nursing finds a unique place in keeping people healthy, holistically intervening to restore health, and enabling the body of Christ and the health care system to work together toward healing.

And Bring Comfort in Suffering and Death

Optimal health means enabling people to live as fully as possible while they are alive. However, despite increasing life spans in many countries, we are mortal beings. The human death rate is still 100 percent. We live in a world that has been corrupted by the effects of sin. Not all of our patients will get well. Some may live with severe physical and mental limitations due to brain damage, loss of limbs, suppressed immune systems or other conditions. Those with degenerative diseases may experience remissions, but the course of the illness causes their bodies, and often their minds, to deteriorate. If health is our only aim in nursing, we can feel only futility and despair in the face of these conditions.

Christian nursing also means providing comfort, hope and compassionate presence for those who are suffering and will not recover. Two hospice nurses explain,

> Caring requires a commitment ... and a willingness to do the unlovely. Neither education nor experience quite prepare you for doing the unlovely.... Caring demands listening and observing with your whole person. ... To care means to be trustworthy. ... Caring is costly. It takes a great amount of physical, emotional, and spiritual energy.[24]

What *does* prepare us for doing the unlovely? How can we keep going when we cannot see physical improvement? Many in our society believe that the answer lies in ending the suffering by terminating life, but Christian nurses are not free to participate in active euthanasia. Only God has the authority to determine when a person should die. We can provide comfort to those who are suffering by keeping them clean, controlling their pain, turning and positioning them. We can advocate for discontinuing futile heroics and unnecessary painful treatments. We can stay with them, surround them with peace and beauty, facilitate relationships with their loved ones, encourage them spiritually and walk with them through the valley of the shadow of death until we must entrust them into the hands of Jesus for the rest of the journey.

In order to provide that kind of care, we need to be walking moment by moment with Jesus ourselves. He is the only one who can prepare us and sustain us in the face of suffering and death. Otherwise they will overcome us. Death is an enemy with deceptive strategies. It tempts us either to seek it (through suicide or euthanasia) or to frantically hold it at bay (through futile heroics or placing hope in miracle cures). Only in Christ can we find realistic hope in the face of suffering and death—and the depth of character needed to provide compassionate accompaniment when hope for recovery is gone.

The Character of the Nurse

Based on the hope given in Christ Jesus and on the presence of the Holy Spirit, Christian nursing should be characterized by love, joy, peace, patience, kindness, goodness, faithfulness, gentleness and self-control (Gal 5:22). This "fruit of the Spirit" results from a dynamic, personal relationship with God through Jesus Christ. We can't work it up on our own. The fruit develops as we put our faith into practice. When we don't feel loving, we act lovingly anyhow. Eventually our feelings may catch up with our actions. Joy and peace don't come naturally, especially in a chaotic working environment where staff do not trust or respect each other. But by focusing on Jesus we can begin to see God at work in difficult situations. Joy and peace grow in the light of eternity. Patience, kindness, goodness, faithfulness, gentleness and self-control sound like characteristics of the ideal nurse. They too come with practice, refined in the furnace of difficult patients, substance-abusing nurse managers, surly nursing assistants, arrogant physicians, and diet kitchens who can't seem to get their orders straight.

Think about the way fruit develops on a tree. It begins as a lovely flower, characteristic of the tree producing it. Soon the blossoms fade, replaced by tiny fruit, which slowly grows larger and sweeter as the tree is nourished by the sun, the rain and the ground. If it is picked prematurely, the fruit will be hard and sour and will not continue to grow. Left to ripen and protected from pests and injury, it will grow until it becomes soft, sweet and nutritious.

Character develops in a similar way. God's Spirit causes "fruit" to blossom and grow in our lives. It is nurtured through prayer, Bible study, worship and Christian fellowship, as well as through practicing being what God intended us to be. At times negative influences in the environment can damage or stunt the growth of the fruit; however, even then there is hope. Some of the best applesauce and apple pies have come from the less-than-perfect apples that dropped from the trees—and next year there will be a new crop. With a little pruning, spraying, fertilizing and watering, the fruit will improve as the trees mature. Eventually we become "like trees planted by streams of water, which yield their fruit in its season" (Ps 1:3).

The common theme in all these aspects of Christian nursing is the glory of God. Nurses, committed to Jesus Christ, holistically caring for the sick, the poor and the needy, demonstrate the character of God to the world. They bring the light of Christ into dark situations with humility, love, passion and power.

Christian nursing is a ministry of compassionate care for the whole person, in response to God's grace toward a sinful world, which aims to foster optimum health (shalom) *and bring comfort in suffering and death for anyone in need.*

14

Spiritual Care

I T WAS THE FIRST SUNDAY OF THE MONTH, AND THE VOLUNTEER parish nurses were taking blood pressures at church after the worship service. Donna lingered in the hall until most of the other people left. Finally she peeked into the room where I (Judy) was putting away my equipment. "I guess I'd better have my blood pressure checked too," she said hesitantly.

Donna, age forty-three, had been coming every month, and I was worried about her. Although she was under medical care and on high doses of medication, her blood pressure stubbornly stayed around 230/120. Married and the mother of four children ranging in age from eighteen down to ten, Donna was grossly overweight and had a different physical ailment every time I saw her.

Accident-prone and highly anxious, she began to tell me that she was sure she would die soon. Her mother had recently been hospitalized with a stroke, and her ninety-three-year-old grandmother had just died of breast cancer. We talked about her fears, then discussed some strategies for reducing her risk of stroke and cancer. But she did not think she could improve her diet or increase her level of activity. She was "too scared" to do breast self-examination or go for a mammogram. She blamed her hypertension and anxiety on her children. Her husband, though faithful, was unsupportive and passive.

Donna teaches kindergarten Sunday school and does an excellent job. She is sensitive to the children, showing particular skill with one autistic child. She vividly conveys God's love to the children, but fears that God is angry with her. Her life feels like it's falling apart. When Donna comes to have her blood pressure checked, she is really seeking spiritual care.

On the other hand, Carol always felt she had her life under control. Bright, capable and on a tenure track at a prestigious university at age twenty-six, she was popular with students and heavily involved with the student Christian fellowship on campus. When she began experiencing severe kidney infections, she followed her medical regimen precisely and fully expected to recover quickly.

Instead, her kidneys shut down permanently, requiring a transplant. All went well for about a year; then her body rejected the kidney. After a second transplant she returned to teaching and working toward her doctorate.

Although Carol lived for another fifteen years, she became acutely aware that her entire body was gradually failing. Finally she admitted that no amount of positive thinking would turn the process around. She called me from her hospital bed, saying, "You know that spiritual care you're always talking about? Well, please come—I need it right now." She died about six months later.

What can nurses offer in the way of spiritual care? In what respect is nursing a Christian ministry?

Probably more than any other profession, nursing deals with giving hope to the hopeless. Although other professionals, such as physicians and clergy, also offer hope, it is the nurse who stands with the sick person for extended periods of time offering care and support when medical science can no longer offer a cure.

Spiritual care must be an integral component of caring for the whole person, and assessing spiritual needs should be included in the total nursing assessment. It is not a nice extra to tack on when we have time, nor should it have to be private and unrecorded. Let's look again at Jesus' approach to the paralytic brought to him by friends:

And just then some people were carrying a paralyzed man lying on a bed. When Jesus saw their faith, he said to the paralytic, "Take heart, son; your sins are forgiven." Then some of the scribes said to themselves, "This man is blaspheming." But Jesus, perceiving their thoughts, said, "Why do you think evil in your hearts? For which is easier, to say, 'Your sins are forgiven,' or to say, 'Stand up and walk'? But so that you may know that the Son of Man has authority on earth to forgive sins"—he then said to the paralytic—"stand up, take your bed and go to your home." And he stood up and went to his home. When the crowds saw it, they were filled with awe, and they glorified God, who had given such authority to human beings. (Mt 9:2-8)

Jesus assessed that although the presenting problem appeared to be physical, the man's primary need at this point was spiritual—forgiveness of sins. Notice that his diagnosis and treatment did not meet with the approval of the community leaders, but he still had the confidence and courage to act on his convictions. Also notice the results. Not only was the man healed, both physically and spiritually, but the crowds glorified God. Good spiritual care should bring glory to God, and not mere comfort to the patient or acceptance with the health care community.

Sometimes spiritual care means simply being present, praying, sharing from Scripture, offering a word of witness and encouragement or participating in a healing service. At other times it may include arranging referrals, planning creative strategies for follow-up care in the home or helping a person become connected to a Christian community.

Myrtle, an eighty-five-year-old in excellent health, never missed a Sunday at church. She sang in the choir, attended a weekly Bible study and served in various volunteer roles with enthusiasm. Then she fell on the ice and broke her arm. Suddenly she became a recluse. Stating that she knew the day would eventually come when she could no longer function and the Lord would take her home, she assumed that that time had now arrived.

When Jean, a nurse from her congregation, visited, she assessed Myrtle's physical needs. More important, she realized that Myrtle had a spiritual need: to know that God still had work for her to do. After listening to Myrtle and praying with her about her concerns, Jean was able to convince Myrtle that a broken arm was hardly life-threatening and she would be able to get out and participate in her activities again. Before long, Myrtle was back at her seat in the choir.

What are spiritual needs? In *Spiritual Care: The Nurse's Role*, Shelly and Fish define a spiritual need as "the lack of any factor or factors necessary to establish and/or maintain a dynamic, personal relationship with God."[1] Although spiritual needs have a horizontal dimension (in relationship to other people), they are primarily vertical (in relationship to God). These include the need for faith, hope and love (1 Cor 13:13), for confession and forgiveness (Jas 5:13-16) and for meaning and purpose (Rom 8:18, Eph 2:10, 3:18-19; Phil 2:13). God meets spiritual needs; we don't. But God works through people, including nurses, to communicate his grace to others. How can nurses provide spiritual care?

Christian spiritual care means facilitating a person's relationship with God through Jesus Christ. That will not always be a "comfort measure." In fact, it may well cause some temporary discomfort as a person becomes aware of sin before a holy God. In our highly secularized postmodern culture, the idea of proclaiming the gospel in a health care setting might seem inappropriate or even impossible; yet, if we truly believe what we claim to believe, salvation through Jesus Christ is the *only* cure for spiritual sickness.

Consider how inappropriate it would be to treat a festering abscess with palliative measures alone. You could give morphine to mask the pain, and the patient would *feel* much better, but the infection would probably keep spreading, causing serious complications and even death. In the same way, offering palliative spiritual interventions without addressing a person's relationship to Jesus Christ will provide only false comfort.

Spiritual care means putting people in touch with God through compassionate presence, active listening, witness, prayer, Bible reading, and partnering with the body of Christ (the church community and the clergy). It is never coercive or rude.

Spiritual care can be appropriate in both secular and Christian settings, and for both Christians and non-Christians. In practical terms spiritual care is usually well received when it is offered in a spirit of gentleness and humility. Christian nurses have often provided spiritual care in secular settings without encountering any resistance from either patients or hospital administration. Sometimes, though, there is opposition.

When patients or family members come from other religious traditions, or no religion, they may refuse any offer of spiritual intervention. Some may request spiritual care from a representative of their own belief system. In such cases we must respect their preferences.

Sometimes that opposition comes when spiritual care is inappropriately offered. I (Judy) once had to fire a nurse who, in addition to providing unsafe physical care, witnessed crassly and manipulatively to her patients. For example, she would ask pre-operative patients, "If you die on the operating table, where will you spend eternity?" Most patients heard nothing beyond the first three words. They refused to sign the operative permits. To this day, I am sure she thinks she was fired for her Christian witness.

Other nurses have been censured for providing good spiritual care. Margie is one example. She was called into the hospital administrator's office and reprimanded for praying with a patient. The administrator learned of this through a glowing letter of appreciation from the patient, who wrote, "The nurses were so caring, especially Margie Johnson, who prayed with me before surgery." He instructed Margie to never pray with a patient again.

Margie belonged to a nurses fellowship group, and she shared her story with them. The group began to pray for the hospital administration. Margie continued to pray with patients when she felt it was appropriate. Within six months the hospital chaplain approached the administrator with a plan for a continuing-education class on spiritual care. He asked Margie to serve on a panel of responders. The administrator attended the event—and was persuaded to change his policy! He began encouraging nurses to provide spiritual care.

Not every story has such a happy ending. Some Christian nurses have continued to work under spiritually oppressive conditions. Others have chosen to change jobs to work in a more open environment. However, our commitment to Christ demands that we remain faithful to him. At times we will need to keep our witness quiet, but we cannot with integrity deny our patients the hope of Jesus Christ because of human rules (Acts 4:19-20; 5:29).

Compassionate Presence

Darryl, thirty-two and dying of AIDS, turned his head toward the window as his evening nurse, Sarah, entered the room. Most of the personnel he had encountered so far seemed distant and subtly contemptuous toward him. The nurse who cared for him on the day shift made such a production of her universal precautions that he knew she was afraid of catching HIV from him. But Sarah seemed different. She laid her hand on his shoulder, saying, "Darryl, you seem tense—would you like a backrub at bedtime?" He relaxed and turned toward her, gratefully accepting the offer.

When the prophet Elijah ran from those who were persecuting him, he became exhausted, depressed and a bit paranoid. God sent an angel, who "touched him" and then told him to "get up and eat" the food prepared for him (1 Kings 19:5). The angel persisted, coming repeatedly, constantly assessing and meeting Elijah's physical, emotional and spiritual needs. The ultimate effect of this angel's intervention was to put Elijah in a position where he could hear personally from God.

In many ways our nursing care is similar to that angel's intervention. We meet patients where they are, provide the assistance needed at the moment and constantly nudge them toward the goals God intends for them. Compassion means to *feel with* another person. Notice, though, that the angel did not stop there. Elijah wanted to die. He felt no hope. The angel did not offer assistance in dying! He came along side Elijah, touched him, allowed him to rest, provided food and water, and sent him on his way when he was sufficiently recovered.

In a similar way Sarah can offer Darryl her compassionate presence: a backrub, feeding him when he is too weak to eat and treating him as the valuable human being that God created him to be. If Darryl receives that kind of humane care, he will be much more open to consider the hope that God has for him in Christ Jesus, and much less compelled to seek assisted suicide.

Active Listening

Nurses have a reputation for being "fixers." When someone suffers, we want to *do something* to ease the pain and provide comfort. Often that response comes in the form of providing answers and solutions, just as Job's friends did. After their harangues, Job called them "miserable comforters" (Job 16:2). He pleaded with them, "Listen carefully to my words. . . . Bear with me and I will speak" (21:2-3). The monologue that followed was not easy to hear. Job complained against God. He spoke in utter despair. But through it all, God was doing an important work in Job's heart. In the end he could affirm, "I had heard of you by the hearing of the ear, but now my eye sees you; therefore I despise myself, and repent in dust and ashes" (42:5-6). Following that confession, Job's life turned around. He regained health, possessions and relationships.

Active listening includes hearing what a person is *not* saying as well as the actual thoughts and feelings articulated. An active listener expresses empathy, humility and commitment to the other, even while sometimes challenging the ideas expressed. Compassionate listening often requires a personal vulnerability that leaves the listener open to rejection or ridicule. We are not talking here about reflective listening, where the nurse stands back and objectively facilitates a verbal catharsis. Instead, we are suggesting an involved dialogue where the nurse enters into the patient's suffering and points the way to hope.

Witness

After careful, active listening, there are times when a word of witness is appropriate and helpful. Ruth Farr used such an approach with a suicidal patient. After carefully assessing the patient through reading her chart, listening and observing, Ruth related:

> In terms of therapeutic communication, I had no idea how to connect with this patient. Nevertheless, the Lord knew how. So it was up to him to provide an opening. If there was something he wanted me to say, I would need his help in knowing the right words to use. In a few minutes he answered my prayer. Her statement "I have to kill myself" was the cue.

"What makes you think you have to kill yourself?" I asked.

"Because I've done so many bad things," she answered.

"But you don't have to die for bad things you've done."

"Yes, I do. I have to be punished. God could never forgive me . . . I'll just have to die."

"But that's why Jesus died for you, so you won't have to die. All you need to do is ask him to forgive you."[2]

Most Christian nurses would not be so bold. Many psychiatric nurses would say that Ruth took a terrible risk by interjecting religious ideation (even though the patient initiated it) and that her solution was too simplistic. But Ruth was apparently listening to the prompting of the Holy Spirit. She clearly documented her intervention. The patient came to a major turning point in her illness, and subsequent nurses notes on the chart by Ruth's colleagues documented the patient's marked improvement.

Sometimes a word of witness can come in the form of a story. The prophet Nathan used that approach with King David after he arranged to have Uriah, the husband of Bathsheba, killed in battle. David had accidentally observed Bathsheba while she was bathing, and he wanted her. Being a man of action, David got what he wanted, and soon Bathsheba gave birth to David's son.

And the LORD sent Nathan to David. He came to him, and said to him, "There were two men in a certain city, the one rich and the other poor. The rich man had very many flocks and herds; but the poor man had nothing but one little ewe lamb, which he had bought. He brought it up, and it grew up with him and with his children; it used to eat of his meager fare, and drink from his cup, and lie in his bosom, and it was like a daughter to him. Now there came a traveler to the rich man, and he was loath to take one of his own flock or herd to prepare for the wayfarer who had come to him, but he took the poor man's lamb, and prepared that for the guest who had come to him." Then David's anger was greatly kindled against the man. He said to Nathan, "As the LORD lives, the man who has done this deserves to die; he shall restore the lamb fourfold, because he did this thing, and because he had no pity."

Nathan said to David, "You are the man!" (2 Sam 12:1-7)

In this case, David responded by immediately confessing his sin and repenting, but he still had to pay the consequences for his behavior. Nathan went on to tell him that the baby would die. When the baby became ill, David fasted and prayed, then fell into a deep depression. It was not until after the baby died that David recovered. If anyone on the scene had been doing research on whether prayer "worked" or measuring the effectiveness of witness as a nursing intervention by whether it produced peace, they would have failed miserably.

A word of witness can also be telling our own stories of how God has met us in difficult time. For example, Cynthia, a nurse who has recovered from breast cancer, visits patients who have been newly diagnosed and leads postmastectomy support groups. She always tells her own story, including how God has helped her through her struggles.

Deirdre is another example. Sexually molested by a male missionary colleague, she has begun to tell her story so that other abused women will find help and hope. Many women who are abused by Christian leaders become disillusioned with the church and may turn away from God and the Christian community. Deirdre's witness affirms God's love in the midst of a horrible experience.

Our witness should not be self-righteous or manipulative, but it can be bold. It includes who God is and what he has done for us in Jesus Christ. More personally, it expresses what God has done in our own lives. It can be very appropriate to humbly share with a patient how God has met us in times of suffering and need. At times when saying "I know what you are going through" does not connect, telling your story can knit a powerful bond and provide hope. It forms a fellowship of suffering that provides strength and encouragement to others who struggle to trust God in hard times. However, whenever we offer a word of witness, we must be sure that it is just that, for when it becomes a sermon it loses its effectiveness.

Prayer—of Many Kinds

Prayer is making big press today. It shows up even in *Time* and *Newsweek*. Nurses, physicians, psychologists and other health care professionals are conducting studies to show that prayer is "good for you" and that prayer "works."[3] Yet on closer observation the prayer being studied scientifically and advocated by everyone from physicians to talk-show hosts looks a lot different from Christian prayer.

Physician and prayer researcher Larry Dossey claims that it really doesn't matter where or to whom we direct our prayers.[4] He prefers to see God as impersonal and refers to him as *the Absolute,* saying,

> The Absolute is radically beyond any description whatsoever, including gender. . . . [T]he reader may insert . . . his or her preferred name for the Absolute—whether *Goddess, God, Allah, Krishna, Brahman, the Tao, the Universal Mind, the Almighty, Alpha and Omega, the One . . .*"[5]

Dossey contends that we should pray because it *works,* not because it maintains our relationship with a loving God. Since research seems to document that prayer is equally effective regardless of to whom it is addressed, he assumes that it really goes nowhere.[6] However, he recognizes a phenomenon of "negative prayer,"[7] while dismissing the reality of the spiritual world.

A quick check of Internet resources on prayer shows 123,530 sites. Limiting the search to healing prayer reduces the number to 38,275.[8] Exploring the web sites uncovers things you never learned in Sunday school—everything from "Angel Answers to Spiritual Questions" (sample answer, "No, Jesus is not part of the Trinity"), "Funky Angel Healing Chakra Doll Prints" (only $2.50 each, in your choice of colors), "HALO Healing Light Order Online Prayer & Healing Ministry" (the URL for "Meet the HALO Team Partners" came up with a blank page), to the more hopeful "Healing Prayer for the Community" (which turned out to be subtitled "Learn Wicca" and included a prayer addressed to the goddess Diana).

What is prayer? Why is it so popular? According to the Bible, prayer is communication with God. Interestingly, there are only 105 references to prayer in the whole Bible (122 to the word *pray*). Jesus taught us how to pray in Matthew 6 by giving the disciples this prayer:

> Pray then in this way: Our Father in heaven, hallowed be your name. Your kingdom come. Your will be done, on earth as it is in heaven.

Give us this day our daily bread. And forgive us our debts, as we also have forgiven our debtors. And do not bring us to the time of trial, but rescue us from the evil one. For if you forgive others their trespasses, your heavenly Father will also forgive you; but if you do not forgive others, neither will your Father forgive your trespasses.(vv. 9-15)

While this prayer asks God for specific things, such as food, forgiveness and protection, its primary focus is on a participation in God's kingdom that requires commitment and action on our part as well.

The Bible *does* tell us that God answers prayer. For example, Matthew 21:22 claims, "Whatever you ask for in prayer with faith, you will receive."

But prayer is not just asking God for things. It also involves praise, adoration, thanksgiving, confession and meditating on God's word. It is the language of relationship, not magic or manipulation.

The first time I (Judy) prayed out loud with a patient was unplanned. In fact, I was fearful of doing the wrong thing. I was a junior nursing student assigned to a seventy-year-old woman who was scheduled for surgery the next day. As I finished her morning care she asked, "Are you a Christian?"

Self-consciously I admitted that I was. We had been sternly warned by our instructors that students were not to discuss religion with patients, and this conversation felt like I might be getting myself into trouble. Then the woman demanded, "Well then, you pray for me!"

I mumbled that I would pray for her when I returned to the dorm that evening.

"No," she responded, "You pray *now, here!*"

I hesitated, pulled the curtain and prayed.

Afterward she was a different person. The once fearful, demanding patient was now hopeful and at peace. When I told my clinical instructor, who was a Christian, about what happened, she personally affirmed me—but reminded me that such behavior was unprofessional.

Is it really appropriate to pray with patients? The obvious answer, if we truly believe that God is our loving Father, is—*of course!* We go to our loving heavenly Father with our concerns for those who are hurting. In so doing we admit our own limitations and acknowledge his love and control of the situation. In the Gospels we see a pattern of just such behavior. The centurion came to Jesus when his servant was sick (Mt 8:5-13), Jairus came on behalf of his daughter (Lk 8). Peter and the other disciples asked Jesus about Peter's mother-in-law's high fever (Lk 4:38). In Luke 9, a father appealed to Jesus for a second opinion after the disciples were unable to heal his son. In Mark 2, a group of friends actually tore the roof off a house in order to bring their paralytic friend to Jesus.

God has told us to come to him with our concerns for the sick and suffering. James writes:

> Are any among you suffering? They should pray. Are any cheerful? They should sing songs of praise. Are any among you sick? They should call for the elders of the church and have them pray over them, anointing them with oil in the name of the Lord. The prayer of faith will save the sick, and the Lord will raise them up; and anyone who has committed sins will be forgiven. Therefore confess your sins to one another, and pray for one another, so that you may be healed. The prayer of the righteous is powerful and effective. (Jas 5:13-16)

Notice here, though, that the One we address in prayer *does* matter. Prayer is more than a technique; it is a relationship with God that is enjoyed at good times as well as in periods of need. Furthermore, this conversation with God is not just a private conversation. It involves the Christian community and the confession of sin within that community. More than a physical cure, healing prayer results in forgiveness of sin and a restoration of relationship with God and his people.

When we pray for our patients, we bring them to the One who created them and loves them, the only One who can truly make them well. Not to do so would be irresponsible. Sometimes we will pray out loud at the bedside, but we should always pray for every patient in our care, even if it is while we walk down the hall to answer a call light, adjust an IV or bathe a comatose patient. Visiting nurses have a wonderful opportunity to pray as they drive. Parish nurses may have the added advantage of a prayer team and healing services.

Bible Reading

The Scriptures can be a deep source of comfort and strength to the believer. The psalmist declares, "Your decrees are my heritage forever; they are the joy of my heart" (Ps 119:111). It is through the Scriptures that we find guidance and direction. Shared appropriately with patients, the Word of God can facilitate powerful spiritual healing.

> Some were sick through their sinful ways, and because of their iniquities endured affliction; they loathed any kind of food, and they drew near to the gates of death. Then they cried to the LORD in their trouble, and he saved them from their distress; he sent out his word and healed them, and delivered them from destruction. (Ps 107:17-20)

On the other hand, the Word of God does spiritual surgery:

> Indeed, the word of God is living and active, sharper than any two-edged sword, piercing until it divides soul from spirit, joints from marrow; it is able to judge the thoughts and intentions of the heart. And before him no creature is hidden, but all are naked and laid bare to the eyes of the one to whom we must render an account. (Heb 4:12-13).

Surgery causes pain before it heals. Sometimes the Bible will confront people with the painful news of their sin before they can hear the good news of salvation. Although we should never use Scripture to blame or attack others, God may well use it to convict people when we read it to them. We cannot measure the effectiveness of our spiritual interventions merely by whether we make patients feel good.

Norma Singer relates an experience where she used the Bible in her nursing care. Alma, a fifty-six-year-old woman admitted to the unit where Norma worked, asked if Norma could stay and talk with her for a few minutes. She poured out her concerns over her complicated medical history and a long list of fears, doubts and guilt. Finally she expressed a fear of dying, because "I don't know what will happen to me!" Norma offered to pray for her, but Alma hesitated, then said, "See, nurse, I had an abortion a long time ago. And I just feel so guilty about it. I guess that's why I don't believe in prayer. Because of what I did."

"Abortion is covered," said Norma.

Then she talked with the surprised woman about God's forgiveness and how even abortion was covered by what Christ did for us on the cross. When a colleague paged Norma, she offered Alma a Bible, pointing out some passages to read about forgiveness. Throughout the day, whenever Norma passed the room she noted that Alma was still reading the Bible. At the end of the shift, Norma again offered to pray with Alma. This time Alma eagerly agreed, and prayed herself, confessing her sin and accepting Christ as Savior.[9]

In this story we see a beautiful example of the Word of God being "living and active" (Heb 4:12). Norma did not have to use it to back up her arguments, convince or coerce Alma. The Bible alone did the work, after Norma's solid groundwork had been laid.

We can use the Bible inappropriately. For example, just quoting our favorite verses without stopping to listen to the patient's concerns will not usually communicate caring or understanding. Too many patients have merely had their suffering compounded by an insensitive Christian who flippantly quoted part of Romans 8:28, "We know that all things work together for good." Furthermore, using the Bible to judge and condemn someone tends to communicate self-righteousness, not hope.

Notice in Norma's story that Alma already felt guilty and assumed God hated her. She needed to hear the good news that God would forgive her, regardless of how bad her sin had been. Reading the Bible convinced her that her sin was indeed covered. Norma's approach took that sin very seriously, but she let God do the judging. The Bible, not Norma, set the standard of righteousness for Alma.

For patients who are already familiar with the Bible, we can often serve them by allowing them to minister to us. Marlene, a visiting nurse, recently related how much she enjoys visiting a particular patient on a weekly basis. Beulah is homebound, but she demonstrates a hopeful attitude and a strong faith. Whenever Marlene visits, Beulah hands her a slip of paper with a Bible verse written on it, saying, "This is your verse for today." Invariably, the verse applies directly to her needs that day.

We can use the same approach with those in our care. A hand-written verse or colorful Bible portion, chosen specifically for an individual patient, will often be carefully read, digested and treasured for years to come. It communicates God's Word, and it also demonstrates our own care and personal interest in the person.

In order to effectively use Scripture in our spiritual care, we need to be familiar with appropriate passages, spend time in personal and group study, and live in daily obedience to what we are learning from the Bible. Setting aside a time for daily personal Bible reading and prayer is essential, even in a hectic schedule. Studying the Bible in a small group provides us with insights from believers. It also gives us the opportunity to practice talking to others about how the Bible applies to daily life, increasing our confidence for sharing with patients. We also need to learn from the experts, including listening to sermons, reading commentaries and books that provide Bible background and application, and perhaps taking courses in Bible and theology.

Functioning as a Body

Partnering with the body of Christ—the church community and the clergy—is another important aspect of spiritual care. Mary Jane, who had been in poor health and homebound for several years, missed her involvement in her church. When nurses from the congregation visited to encourage her and to assess her changing needs, Mary Jane expressed frustration that she could not get out to church activities.

So the nurses brought the church to Mary Jane. She became the official volunteer coordinator, each week calling every person who had a part in the upcoming Sunday services, from children's choir members to ushers. She also initiated the congregation's prayer chain, catalogued books for the church library and made crafts for special occasions. Mary Jane probably knew more about what was happening in the church than any of those who attended regularly. Her involvement with the church met a spiritual need for Christian community.

We are created in God's image, which means we are designed to live in relationship with God and with one another. We need the body of Christ, the church, in order to live healthy lives. When a person becomes institutionalized or homebound, the isolation from the church compounds the sense of brokenness. An important aspect of spiritual care is connecting our patients to the Christian community.

While visiting Korea we were amazed at how seriously the Korean churches take this responsibility. One Christian hospital in particular is surrounded by dozens of churches started for the express purpose of incorporating all the new Christians who came to know the Lord through the ministry of that hospital. Nurses can provide only a small, though significant, part of the whole spectrum of spiritual care. For the most part that care will come through the church.

We can begin to connect patients with the church by asking whether they are associated with a church and whether their pastor knows about their present condition. Has their pastor, deacon, parish nurse or other member of their congregation visited recently? If not, would they appreciate it if a family member or the nurse notified the pastor about any important changes in their health status?

Recently Martha, an active member of my (Judy's) congregation who lived alone, became seriously ill. She panicked and called an ambulance but did not tell anyone in the church, because she was too weak to make any more phone calls and too embarrassed to bother anyone. The effective grapevine of a small community, along with the prompting of the Holy Spirit, finally got the word to the pastor and to me. A neighbor saw the ambulance and called a church member the next day. That woman tried calling Martha at home. When she got no answer, she began calling local hospitals until she located Martha, then called the pastor to report. The pastor and I visited Martha in the hospital, and she deeply appreciated the time of fellowship and prayer and felt relieved that we could notify her friends and extended family.

Our visit also drew in Martha's hospital roommate, Eunice, who was also a Christian. We ended up all joining hands and praying together. Up to that point Martha and Eunice had not talked about their faith with one another. Following the visit, they began praying together.

Intentionally including the pastor and the church community in the health care team may facilitate the healing process. Recent nursing literature has begun to recognize the importance of the church community in health care.[10] In many cases, the church is merely viewed as another community-based location for primary health care. However, even when the spiritual dimension of care is limited, patients may perceive the care they receive as more caring and holistic. Frank is a good example.

Another long-time member of our church and an adult-onset diabetic, Frank at age eighty had little interest in following a diabetic diet. He would fast before going for his blood glucose tests, but he ate whatever he wanted in between. I had noticed that his general health seemed to be deteriorating. When the parish nurses at church sponsored a health fair in conjunction with the annual bazaar, I convinced Frank to come in to get his blood sugar tested. It was 542 mg./dl. We called his physician, who met him at the hospital emergency room. By the time Frank arrived at the hospital, his blood sugar was well over 600 mg./dl. His wife called me when they got home and reported that Frank had finally decided to take his diet seriously. "He wouldn't listen to me, but he is listening to you now," she remarked. Frank continues to check in periodically to tell me how his blood sugar is doing and assure me that he is sticking to his diet. In Frank's case there was little overt spiritual care offered. However, because we worship together and have a long-term friendship, Frank trusts me with his physical health.

Another way the church meets our patients' spiritual needs is through the sacraments. The Lord's Supper was intended to be a healing event, a celebration of Christian unity and the salvation provided in the death and resurrection of Jesus Christ. As such, we can call on the clergy to bring the sacrament of communion to those in our care. However, the Lord's Supper is not magic and should never be offered lightly.

The sacraments, according to the *Book of Common Prayer*, are "an outward and visible sign of an inward and spiritual grace given unto us; ordained by Christ himself, as a means by whereby we receive the same, and a pledge to assure us thereof."[11] Augustine of Hippo defined them as "a visible sign of an invisible reality."[12]

Augustine categorized around thirty liturgical ceremonies as sacraments.[13] By the Middle Ages the church had distinguished seven: baptism, confirmation, communion, marriage, penance, extreme unction and ordination. Catholics churches still recognize all seven. Most Protestant churches recognize two sacraments: baptism and communion (or the Lord's Supper). Except for baptism in the case of imminent death, most churches require ordained clergy to preside over the sacraments. However, nurses can be alert for appropriate opportunities to facilitate bringing clergy into the health care team so that the sacraments can be offered.

Supportive Presence

We cannot underestimate the power of supportive presence in spiritual care—what Luther called the "mutual consolation of the saints." This involves active listening, encouragement, expressing faith and hope—and physical care. Anticipating a person's physical needs, being willing to cheerfully handle foul-smelling excrement and bodily discharges, offering a gentle touch or a helping hand, all communicate personal dignity and worth. They are just as much spiritual care as prayer and Bible reading. Perhaps one of the strongest drawing points of many alternative therapies is that practitioners spend extended time with the patient, paying particular attention to the body. However, only in the biblical worldview is the physical body viewed as reflecting the image of God and thereby worthy of respect and care.

Spiritual care is not a set of techniques, although we have many resources at our disposal. Spiritual care is a way of life that involves walking together with the Lord. Sometimes it is merely a listening ear or a gentle touch. At other times it requires confrontation. The basic resources we have to offer are prayer, the Word of God and the Christian community; however, the most important resource is God himself. The ultimate aim of our spiritual care is to bring people into dynamic personal relationship with Jesus Christ and the fellowship of his people.

15

Looking
to the Future

THE NURSES' STATION BUZZED WITH ACTIVITY. THIS SHIFT had gone from hectic to chaotic as the day progressed. Patients returning from the recovery room seemed sicker than usual, requiring extra time and attention. Six physicians sat at the desk writing orders, tossing charts into precarious piles. Call lights seemed to be flashing from every room. In the midst of this pandemonium, the elevator doors flew open and spewed out Dr. Devine, pushing a stretcher bearing an ashen, moaning woman.

"I want my patient transferred to this floor immediately!" he roared. The nurses on the unit had always joked that Dr. Devine took his name seriously—he thought he was God.

Gingerly I (Judy) replied, "Dr. Devine, we can't do that. Only the admissions office can transfer patients between units. Besides, every bed is full."

After a tirade of obscenities, he finally settled down and explained, "Patients on this floor get well faster. You're good nurses. I want my patient to have the best."

What qualities did Dr. Devine see in our nursing care? He never really elaborated, and he may not have even known what made the difference—

except that his patients seemed to get well faster. What makes a *good nurse?* In a time of rapidly changing roles and expectations, is there anything that remains constant in the definition of a good nurse? Perhaps another story will illustrate one of those constants.

Standing in line while waiting to enter a theater, I (Judy) heard a voice calling, "Nurse! Nurse!" and saw a woman I did not recognize rushing toward me with a man in tow. When they arrived at my side, she said to the man, "This is my nurse!" Then she turned to me and explained apologetically, "I wanted my husband to meet you." She continued to her husband, "She's a good nurse. She brought me warm milk when I couldn't sleep, and then she prayed with me." At that point I remembered her. I had cared for her postoperatively over a year before.

Actually, this woman had been a rather difficult patient, not only due to her anxiety and insomnia, but because her condition initially required a great deal of complicated care. She had tested my nursing skills to the maximum. The warm milk and bedtime prayer offered the night before her discharge seemed insignificant to me compared with managing all the treatments, medications, tubes and wires earlier in her hospitalization. Why did she view them as the mark of a good nurse?

In the survey of Christian nurses described in chapter one we asked, *What characteristics do nurses need most?* Compassion rated highest (listed by 80 percent of participants), followed by competence (52 percent), faith commitment (26 percent), integrity (25 percent) and responsibility (10 percent).[1]

Scottish nurse educator Annette Morrison writes, "Indeed, I would suggest to you that we are now witnessing an almost universal appeal by nurses worldwide to return to the basic traditional skills of nursing that uniquely identify the 'caring nature' of the nurse as perceived by the public in general."[2]

As we face the implications of managed care, most nurses feel that we are losing something extremely important in nursing. The core of our identity seems to be eroding at the expense of cost effectiveness. Furthermore, Bishop and Scudder contend that "professionalization may be obscuring the moral sense of nursing."[3] Jesus set the moral standard for nursing by telling the story of the good Samaritan. That standard is no less than compassion—a compassion that demands competent care, given with commitment to the patient, integrity and a deep sense of responsibility.

What will nursing look like throughout the twenty-first century? Economics will continue to shape health care delivery. The specific tasks may change. Technological developments will continue to escalate. The milieu may be radically different. Nursing, however, will continue to be a ministry of compassionate health care to anyone in need. The mark of a good nurse will always be compassion—offering that cup of cold water (or warm milk) in the name of the Lord.

Nursing's Expanding Context

We have demonstrated throughout this book that nursing must view the person as holistic—a biopsychosocial unity. That concept is not unique to Christian nursing. Have you ever met a nurse who saw only the physical aspect of care as defining nursing? We all know that when a person is hurting emotionally, all sorts of physical ailments crop up. On the other hand, physical conditions can affect the mind and the spirit. It's hard to concentrate or pray when you're hurting. Alzheimer's destroys the body and the mind. A diagnosis of serious illness may cause a person to give up hope and die.

We have also examined the biblical understanding of *shalom* as it relates to health. Individuals, created by God with unique value and worth, find fulfillment in relationship with a human community. Most nurses today also acknowledge that we care for individuals in the context of families and communities. However, few have stopped to consider the full implications of that understanding. Of course we support the family members who are present with our patients, we tap into community resources, and perhaps we even include their clergy in our care plans, but there is a larger perspective. Human connections—like families, communities and churches—function together to facilitate health. Nursing practice in the future will expand to include a broader participation in these extended relationships.

First Corinthians 12:12-31 provides us with a glimpse at how God uses these interconnections. We are to be the body of Christ. Each organ functions uniquely, and they all need each other. Hearts can't do much good without lungs. Our bodies need nutrients digested and waste products excreted to sustain life. In a similar way God puts individuals into relationships. For Christians, a primary connection is the church. Within the church we support and care for one another. We can't just amputate a body part when it gives us trouble without affecting the whole body. When one part hurts, we all suffer. When one part receives honor, we all share in the glory.

The context of the church as a center for health care will continue to expand as economically driven health systems leave people confused and underserved. Nurses will be involved through counseling, leading support groups, teaching wellness, training lay caregivers, establishing and running centers for primary health care, referring people to appropriate resources and advocating for them in the health care system. We may even need to come full circle and again start establishing church-owned and operated hospitals and extended-care facilities.

Nurses will also be involved in supporting families. None of these families is perfect. The first dysfunctional family appeared soon after creation, and they passed on their destructive family processes to all the generations that followed. Read the book of Genesis if you want to see the problem dramatically illustrated. However, the family is still the best place to find the love and nurture we need to prepare us for life. We then move out of our families of origin into new families, churches and communities, only to re-enact the same old patterns—both positive and negative.

As nurses we have the advantage of recognizing some of the dynamics involved in human relationships. To some degree we can be objective observers of the interrelationships between those processes. The skills we have learned in assessment, planning, intervention and evaluation serve us well as we move into a new era of health care with shifting values, goals and areas of practice. We are living in a time of increasingly broken relationships. The pain experienced in unstable families spills over into the church, the workplace and the community at large. As nurses we have some important contributions to make toward health and healing in each of these systems. For example, we can use our nursing skills to change unhealthy patterns in family dynamics through providing education and support for single parents, substance abusers and those affected by chronic illness or grief.

As we move into the ever-expanding contexts of nursing—often not by our own choosing—we need to remember the biblical injunction, "Since we are surrounded by so great a cloud of witnesses, let us also lay aside every weight and the sin that clings so closely, and let us run with perseverance the race that is set before us, looking to Jesus the pioneer and perfecter of our faith" (Heb 12:1-2). The race is not easy. Listen to the voices of three discouraged nurses:

I wish I could see the opportunity and not just crises. I think I'm too cynical just now to be positive about nursing. I do believe I have expertise to offer patients. The longer I'm at this agency (reputedly the best in the area to work for) the more I think some portion of my frustration is the attitude there. I'm always better off when I try to avoid the office. But the flip side of that is loneliness. This is a pretty lonely job.—*a home care nurse in New York*

The small-town hospital that I have grown to love, and the fourth floor that I think of as my home and family, is going through so many changes. I go to work and don't recognize it anymore, and soon they will be dismantling us as a unit. I see my floor dying. I find little hope that this latest change is for the good of the patients and the staff. I come home at night feeling totally defeated.—*a hospital staff nurse in Massachusetts*

I quit my job, finally, after twenty-seven years! It was with a great deal of sadness and regret that I finally threw in the towel. So much has happened to bring that about. Everything's changing so much in nursing I wasn't really enjoying it anymore. I tried so hard to weather every storm and then finally saw that I couldn't keep up with it, that some of the changes were compromising me professionally, not to mention short-changing the patients. And so, it seemed like a good time to make my exit. I can't tell you how hard it was to walk away from all that need, though. But you can't serve two masters, even two that you love, and I knew the time had come to make a choice.—*a hospital staff nurse in Illinois*

Maintaining Integrity in Nursing Practice
All of these nurses are Christians who sincerely want to serve God and care

for people. One has quit; the other two hang on but wonder how much longer they can do it. In the midst of this general sense of discouragement in nursing however, some bright glimmers of hope continue to appear. Recently the *Journal of Christian Nursing* put out a call for brief articles on "Why I Love Nursing." The response was enthusiastic. What made these nurses different from their dispirited colleagues? Three common themes seemed to ring out from each of these authors: a sense of serving God by what they were doing, joy in their interpersonal relationships, and an ability to see the big picture.

First, their *sense of serving God* gave these nurses a vision of a greater mission and a willingness to suffer for it. This theme is perhaps most strongly voiced by those serving through their churches as parish nurses or congregational health ministers. Over and over, these nurses exclaim, "This is what I came into nursing to do!" Many of them have quit high-paying jobs in secular nursing to work for little or no pay. What are they doing? Health assessments, screening, teaching, counseling, praying—and encouraging people to see the connection between faith and health.

On the other hand, many nurses are sensing God's call within their secular jobs. A home health nurse recently wrote, "God has given me a burden for the inner-city mother. I have just begun to keep a journal of my encounters." She has every reason to be discouraged. Her agency has faced all the upheaval and distress that managed care delivers. She has already lost one job to an agency closure. Her present clientele are the poorest of the poor. Their problems seem insurmountable. But God has given her a burden for these people, and she's writing it down. Where that will lead she doesn't know yet.

In a culture raised on a false gospel of "health and wealth," most of us have difficulty seeing God's hand in situations that involve pain, suffering and deprivation. Some would go so far as to say that God is not blessing us if we must suffer loss or even discomfort. The apostle Paul had a different perspective. In writing to the Corinthian church he explained:

> For it is the God who said, "Let light shine out of darkness," who has shone in our hearts to give the light of the knowledge of the glory of

God in the face of Jesus Christ.

But we have this treasure in clay jars, so that it may be made clear that this extraordinary power belongs to God and does not come from us. We are afflicted in every way, but not crushed; perplexed, but not driven to despair; persecuted, but not forsaken; struck down, but not destroyed; always carrying in the body the death of Jesus, so that the life of Jesus may also be made visible in our bodies. For while we live, we are always being given up to death for Jesus' sake, so that the life of Jesus may be made visible in our mortal flesh. (2 Cor 4:6-11)

Although nursing in recent years has been viewed as a fairly high-paying, secure job, we have seen in earlier chapters that it did not begin that way. Throughout history nurses have viewed their work as a calling from God, and they have entered into the suffering of others to make a difference. To do that means challenging the forces of sin and evil in the world in the name of Jesus. Of course there will be opposition! The way will not be easy. But we will find a keen sense of mission and direction from God that gives us the hope to keep going when we feel afflicted, perplexed, persecuted and struck down.

A second common thread in the testimonies of nurses who love nursing is a *delight in interpersonal relationships with patients and colleagues.* There is a deep sense of compassion for those who are suffering, an entering into their lives to comfort and to care. These nurses tell stories of patients who got better against all odds, and others who died in peace, because of the nursing care they received. They relate incidents where they were able to help a colleague out of a tough situation or enable a health care team to work together in harmony. They also tell about how patients and coworkers encouraged them. That sense of mutuality makes them want to go to work each day, even in the midst of organizational change and personal injustices.

This same sense of joy inspired Paul in tough times. Consider 1 Thessalonians 2:19: "For what is our hope or joy or crown of boasting before our Lord Jesus at his coming? Is it not you?" The work he invested in the Thessalonian believers was rewarded as he saw their spiritual growth.

In the same way, we find joy and worth in our work by seeing patients get well or die peacefully, and by working with a team that supports and respects one another. Paul continues in 1 Thessalonians 3:9: "How can we thank God enough for you in return for all the joy that we feel before our God because of you?" Seeing the fruit of our labors gives us the encouragement to keep going when the way becomes difficult.

The third common thread among nurses who love nursing is an *ability to see the big picture*. When crisis hits, they do not focus on what they are losing—they consider the needs and opportunities that arise out of the situation. They are willing to change and to take risks. Sometimes this means going back to school, moving to another area of nursing (or another location) or even breaking out into a completely new venture. These nurses have started nurse-managed clinics, extended-care facilities and consultant services. Some have gone overseas as missionaries. Others have created new roles such as "spiritual care specialist" or "parish nurse coordinator" within their present institutions.

A hospital staff nurse in Ohio writes, "I have chosen my goal—to serve Christ as a nurse. This has become my way of life, my ideal. I have a vision of the kind of nurse I want to be and I have the motivation I need—Christ. I am learning to trust him to help me achieve." She became a nurse after twenty years as a respiratory therapist. She knew that she might not find a job in nursing when she graduated, but she persevered because she knew God was calling her.

A home health nurse in California saw people in her community falling through the cracks of the health care system, while at the same time several Christian nurses in her congregation lost their jobs due to downsizing. She worked with them to set up a Christian home care agency that provides care at affordable rates.

Again we turn to the apostle Paul, who writes:

Not that I have already obtained this or have already reached the goal; but I press on to make it my own, because Christ Jesus has made me his own. Beloved, I do not consider that I have made it my own; but this one thing I do: forgetting what lies behind and straining forward to what lies ahead, I press on toward the goal for the prize of the heavenly call of God in Christ Jesus. (Phil 3:12-14)

The goal of nursing is not personal satisfaction; it is not maintaining the health care system as we have known it in the past few decades. Christian nursing has always been about pressing on toward the heavenly call of God in Christ Jesus—working toward *shalom*, announcing the in-breaking kingdom of God and demonstrating its presence through acts of justice and mercy. When we keep this goal in mind we can look ahead with expectancy, knowing that when God calls us he will lead us and ultimately work things together for good (Rom 8:28).

The Changing Face of Nursing Education

"I feel so guilty teaching students when we are preparing them for jobs that won't exist when they graduate," a nursing instructor recently confessed.

As nursing practice changes, so must nursing education. Central to the task of nursing education is the need to clearly envision the knowledge and skills that will equip today's students to be tomorrow's practitioners. However, rather than looking at fads and trends, we have attempted to reexamine the nursing metaparadigm from an eternal perspective—to develop a theology of nursing. In doing so we hope to gain insight into the trends and discernment over the fads.

It is God who calls us into nursing in the first place and gives us the wisdom and strength to endure when the going gets tough. Nursing education that neglects teaching this perspective leaves students without a moral foundation or clear motivation for nursing.

Nursing theory development is essentially a theological as well as philosophical process. So is curriculum development. Without a solid understanding of who God is and what he intends for us to be, we cannot develop appropriate nursing curricula or design strong courses to prepare future nurses. Part of the root cause of nursing's present confusion—and to a large degree, disintegration—comes from the absence of a guiding common theology. Some are trying to superimpose three opposing paradigms and come up with an "inclusive" whole. Others pick and choose eclectically, supposing that they can merely take what seems best from each. That simply won't work.

As we have seen, many of the current health care fads draw nurses toward occult practices and idolatry. Shifting moral values and ethical approaches, alternative therapies, new paradigms and expanded roles lure nurses into seemingly attractive directions. Only a clear understanding of Christian theology, along with a vital faith relationship with God, will give us the discernment to choose wisely and faithfully from the increasing array of options available.

Furthermore, students need to gain competence in practical theology—knowing how to share their faith, how to pray with patients and read Scripture appropriately, how to listen to the Spirit as well as the patient, and how to participate as colleagues in ministry along with the clergy and the body of Christ. Even students with strong personal faith need to learn how to practice Christian ministry in a health care setting.

The need for a theological foundation for nursing becomes especially evident in parish nursing or congregational health ministry. Those who teach parish nurses must be well grounded in theology as well as nursing. A nurse educator who happens to be a Christian is no more prepared to teach parish nursing than a theologian who makes occasional hospital visits. However, most parish-nurse education programs are currently taught by a combination of nurses and theologians who are not adequately prepared in both disciplines. We need a growing number of nurse-theologians who can view nursing through the eyes of faith, not only to teach parish nurses but to shape the future of nursing and nursing education.

Revisiting the Nursing Metaparadigm

Once we have established a theological focus, nursing education needs to take seriously the biblical view of the person, the environment and health. Several themes require special consideration: the goodness of creation, the effects of sin, the seen and the unseen aspects of the environment, the mandate God has given us as caretakers of creation, and the understanding of the person as an integrated whole, created to live in *shalom* with God, the human community and the environment.

Mary Oesterle and Darlene O'Callaghan outline some of the big questions in nursing education today:

1. In a health care system that is increasingly defining roles and responsibilities of assistive personnel, are basic skills such as bed-bath and bed-making principles essential content to a baccalaureate curriculum?

2. Why are we preparing students with an emphasis on practice in acute-care hospitals when the futurists identify them as becoming a collection of intensive care units, employing a limited number of our graduates?

3. Is nursing education congruent with the needs of the emerging health care environment?

4. Can we afford to structure our curriculum around specific content when knowledge changes so rapidly?

5. Why do we continue this focus on skills when assessment knowledge, critical thinking, decision-making, and collaboration are essential processes of the future?[4]

It is in response to these questions that a biblical view of the nursing metaparadigm gives profound insight. Let's look at the first question. Yes the reality for nursing today is that assistive personnel will be performing most of the physical care in the community as well as in acute-care settings. Many skills will become obsolete. Who needs mitered corners when we have fitted sheets? On the other hand, how many nursing students today have ever learned to make a bed properly? Can they teach the assistive personnel? Can they look at a patient and figure out that the decubitus on his sacrum may have something to do with lumps in the linens and improper positioning? Will they even see the bedsore if they do not spend time assessing the patient's skin while performing a bedbath?

Consider the perspective given by nurse educator Carol Bence as she addresses her graduating class:

When we bathe another person we cross the intimacy barrier; something is shared. We get up close and personal with another human being. We enter his or her world. It is a humbling act for both the washer and the washee. It is an act of compassion. Too often, perhaps, we want to hurry through the bath so we can get on with the more important aspects of nursing. But perhaps it is in the simple ritual of the bath that we discover what it means to be a true nurse.[5]

As Christians we have a unique understanding of and respect for the human body. Our theology tells us that the body is important, warranting our nurture and care. In our rush to prepare managers and health promoters, we dare not neglect the seemingly mundane details of physical care.

In relating to assistive personnel Christian nurses have a model of servant leadership in Jesus Christ. Rather than seeking glory in the "more important roles" of the professional nurse, we have a responsibility to respect and support assistive personnel. If we really care for patients, then we must also care for those who are providing the front-line patient care. We also need to give them good reason to respect us by demonstrating competency, confidence and compassion.

To answer Oesterle and O'Callaghan's second question, no, we do not want to prepare nurses who are primarily oriented to acute care; however, we must be careful not to assume that students will be able to gain confidence in nursing skills and see the whole picture of health care without experience in a hospital setting. Many of the skills now required in home care and extended-care facilities were formerly practiced only in hospitals. That trend will probably continue. The hospital provides a safer environment for students to learn the principles behind the skills that will transfer later into other situations and specific applications. The hospital also affords the student a community of mentors who can model safe, ethical care, and a backup system when they fail.

Nursing education will have to change to meet the needs of the emerging health care environment. Students will need to have creative community experience to gain and apply expertise in assessment, critical thinking, decision-making and collaboration. Yet there must always be a body of knowledge and skill that makes a nurse a nurse. Of course skills will change! Most of the nursing skills we learned as nursing students are obsolete—dissolving morphine in sterile spoons for injection, sharpening needles, constructing chest suction with rubber tubes and glass bottles, even reading the mercury in thermometers and sphygmomanometers. But the principles involved were easily transferable to new technologies.

As we consider the legitimate questions that must be raised about how students are prepared for nursing in the next decade, we must continue to focus our attention on what makes nursing *nursing*. Obviously it is not specific skills, a particular context or even an immutable body of knowledge. We have defined Christian nursing as *a ministry of compassionate care for the whole person, in response to God's grace toward a sinful world, which aims to foster optimum health* (shalom) *and bring comfort in suffering and death for anyone in need*. The way we prepare nursing students must include the best of science, technology, the arts and practical skills, which are consistent with a Christian worldview in order to nurture people toward health.

In the process we must not lose sight of the whole person or any dimensions of that wholeness. We must not neglect the care of the body or the care of the soul. We must also be careful to maintain *shalom*, for those in our care and all those within the nursing community. We must guard against preparing nurses to be lone practitioners without the support and accountability of a professional community as well as a Christian community.

Finally, we must keep our focus on those qualities that make a *nurse*. While critical thinking, decision-making and leadership skills are extremely important, our research shows that practicing nurses believe that the characteristics nurses need most are compassion, competence, faith, integrity and responsibility. Those values are consistent with what Jesus requires of us. In Matthew 22:37-39 Jesus tells us: " 'You shall love the Lord your God with all your heart, and with all your soul, and with all your mind.' This is the greatest and first commandment. And a second is like it: 'You shall love your neighbor as yourself.' "

One of the greatest challenges for nursing education in the coming years will be shaping the character of students who have grown up in a culture that cripples them in three ways:

□ They have been given no standard of absolute truth.

□ They have few models of love and faithfulness.

□ They have absorbed a sense of personal entitlement that views selfless care for others as dysfunctional behavior.

Nursing must return to its theological roots to maintain its heart and soul.

Exploring the Challenge Before Us: Nursing Research

Ever since nursing education entered the university through the door of science, nursing educators have been working to establish a body of knowledge unique to nursing through research. As we saw in chapter two, this orientation became the impetus for developing nursing theories. Most of the earlier nursing theories reflect the influence of naturalistic science. Because such theories could not adequately account for the human experience of health and illness, nurses broadened the scope of nursing theory. Inevitably such theories have moved into areas traditionally viewed as religious, although they are often called scientific to maintain credibility in the university. Research moved from the quantitative and objective to a more qualitative and subjective mode.

Nurses doing nursing research need to be clear about the philosophical and theological underpinnings of the theories they use. Under pressure to complete theses and dissertations, Christian nurses often select research instruments without a clear understanding of their underlying philosophies. Such instruments are not neutral. The questions, and the things they are designed to measure, contain worldview and religious assumptions that need to be discerned and explicitly described.

Many who use qualitative approaches such as grounded theory and phenomenology assume that they can approach the research situation without being influenced by their own beliefs. Rather than forcing the data into a preconceived mold, they believe truth emerges from the situation itself. The attempt to learn from the situation and from our patients is admirable. But researchers cannot free themselves of their own theological or philosophical assumptions. This is a good thing, for it is through the dialogue between our experience and our prior beliefs that we build our knowledge base. What keeps this dialogue from merely going in circles, for Christians, is that we can test our conclusions by God's revelation to us in Scripture. This is particularly important in studies involving psychosocial and spiritual concepts. Nurse researchers need to recognize their own presuppositions in order to be fair to those who read and use their work.

Good research will help nurses to improve patient care. All aspects of the person are legitimate areas for research—physical, emotional and psychological, social and spiritual. The increasing interest in spirituality and health carries both positive and negative connotations, however. As we have seen, Christian spirituality concerns the relationship of people with God. Using God as a means to improved health, however, is actually a form of idolatry. Research studies designed to show the correlation between health and religious practices such as prayer and church attendance are legitimate, so long as they are presented only as descriptions of what people do and how they respond, not what God does. Positive correlations *may* indicate what *generally* is the case for people who love and obey God.

Studies about prayer can be viewed only from the human side. God, by his very nature, cannot be locked into a cause-and-effect study. Further, most studies purporting to show the value of prayer do not make any claims about the kind of god being addressed. Most of them simply account for any benefits on the basis of the psychological effect of ritual. Some researchers, however, consider prayer a means of linking into the universal consciousness. Christians who want to study any relationship between prayer and health must use a biblical definition of prayer.

Research studies on spiritual needs of patients abound. Usually patients are asked what they see as their spiritual needs. In other instances nurse researchers use questionnaires with built-in assumptions about the nature of spiritual needs. In both approaches the identified spiritual needs may not be the real needs of patients. For example, the Bible has much to say about godly sorrow and repentance from sin. Repentance and sin are not the focus of nursing studies. In fact, most studies of spiritual needs deal mainly with patients' psychology and say little or nothing about a relationship between God and the person. Christians need to come to their research with a biblical understanding of the spiritual.

As nurses we must never lose our concern for patients' physical well-being. Research on physical outcomes of nursing care is still needed, especially with the onset of managed care. Good research can help us to recommend appropriate standards for care to health care agencies and insurance companies.

Finally, Christian nurses must be humble about their findings. We know that the full meaning of being human cannot be captured in research. The person, the environment, health and nursing can be understood only in relationship with God. Discovering the fullness and the implications of that relationship is a lifelong process. In fact, it cannot fully be accomplished in this life. In the meantime, we walk in faith.

A Practical Theology

Once, when asked to summarize his theology, the eminent theologian Karl Barth replied, "Jesus loves me, this I know, for the Bible tells me so." In the face of a complicated technological society and an uncertain future, we might do well to stick with such a basic assertion. God's love, demonstrated for us in the person of Jesus Christ and recorded in the Bible, certainly provides the core of our theological stance.

Because God's love is active and empowering, our theology must also be practical and dynamic. In nursing, knowing God's love impels us to care for anyone in need, as it has always inspired nurses in the past. Nursing demonstrates God's love in a ministry of compassionate care for the whole person—physical, psychosocial and spiritual. It aims to foster optimum health and bring comfort in suffering and death. The health toward which we strive is part of the greater work of God in his people to bring completeness, soundness and well-being *(shalom)* to the total person—in relationship to God, self, others and the environment. Nursing is a work of God's grace. We are privileged to share in that work.

Appendix

Guidelines for Evaluating Alternative Therapies

T HE FOLLOWING QUESTIONS CAN BE GUIDELINES FOR EVALU-
ating holistic health modalities. They provide us with a systematic way to
assess the potential religious and philosophical problems hiding behind
alternative therapies.[1]

Modality

1. What techniques are necessary to practice the modality (meditation,
"centering," mind control and so on)? Meditating on a portion of Scripture
or the character of God may be helpful; emptying the mind, or using Eastern
techniques, can be dangerous.

2. Are assumptions made regarding human nature or the nature of
ultimate reality? If so, are they compatible with Scripture? Techniques that
purport to manipulate energy often explain it as being the Holy Spirit.
Remember, the Holy Spirit is *God*, and we cannot manipulate God; instead,
we must obey him.

3. Are these assumptions clearly evident to all observers, or must one be
involved with the modality to determine what they are? Most alternative
therapies are experientially based. Spiritual assumptions will not be evident
until after a person has practiced them for a while. However, nursing

literature is expressing these assumptions more overtly as public acceptance increases.

4. Has the technique been subjected to peer-reviewed scientific research, and have results been confirmed by subsequent studies? Keep in mind that poor research can prove almost anything. Some alternative therapies are based only on anecdotal evidence.

5. What is the level of intervention (e.g., etiology, symptom relief)? Does it merely serve to make the person feel good temporarily? Might it mask symptoms that need urgent medical attention?

Practitioner

1. What is the practitioner's worldview? Does he or she try to persuade clients to accept this worldview? In 2 Corinthians 4:2 Paul says, "We have renounced the shameful things that one hides; we refuse to practice cunning or to falsify God's word; but by the open statement of the truth we commend ourselves to the conscience of everyone in the sight of God." There is a big difference between surreptitious persuasion and true evangelism—which is essentially telling the good news about Jesus without manipulation or deceit.

2. Does the practitioner claim a particular source of power? If so, is it compatible with Christian belief? A colleague recently attended a continuing nursing education program, approved by the state nurses association, where the instructor claimed that her content on "healing touch" had been channeled to her by a spirit guide. If supernatural powers are involved here, they are evil ones.

3. Does the practitioner demonstrate an awareness of possible underlying religious assumptions and their implications? For example, nursing theorist Jean Watson appeals to pre-Christian Scandinavian runic tradition (among other religious influences), saying of her trip to Sweden, "Consulting the runes literally or metaphorically starts my journey of remembering, because runic consciousness enables me to bypass the structures of reason, the fetters of conditioning and the momentum of habit and experience a more true present—the now that makes me more malleable, vulnerable, and open to change."[2]

Client

1. Does practicing the modality require a change in lifestyle? If so, does the change appear to be positive or negative? Is the change compatible with Christian beliefs? Changes might include meditation techniques, arranging furniture to facilitate the proper flow of energy, nutritional adaptations (e.g., eating a balance of "hot" and "cold" foods), withdrawing from personal relationships, joining a community and participating in its group rituals, or following a certain spiritual teacher.

2. Does health improve; is suffering relieved? To what extent? For how long? Although effectiveness holds a powerful attraction, it should not be the only criterion. Many things that make us feel good are not good for us.

3. Are there any short- or long-term adverse side effects (physically, mentally or spiritually)? Hillstrom throws some interesting light on the benefits of Eastern meditation. She describes research studies indicating that there is no difference between the brain waves of people who are meditating and those who are merely resting or sleeping. She continues, "Significantly, there are also studies indicating that Eastern-style meditation can have adverse and long-lasting physical and psychological consequences." These effects include headaches, insomnia, gastrointestinal upsets, anxiety, depression, confusion, mental and physical tension and inexplicable outbursts of antisocial behavior.[3]

Numerous meditators have themselves told us that entering into meditation without a spiritual guide is dangerous because of the physical and psychological side effects. Christians who attempt these meditative techniques often report an inability to pray or comprehend the Bible.

Results

1. What is the stated explanation for the results?

2. Is the explanation generally accepted by health professionals, or is it subject to controversy?

3. Do the explanations for the results seem to contradict scriptural teaching in any way?

4. What are other possible explanations?

Notes

Chapter 1: Caring & the Christian Story

[1]Christine Ann Grem, "Cameo of Caring: George," *Journal of Christian Nursing,* summer 1995, p. 9.

[2]Rosene M. Dunkle, "Beyond Appearances: Caring in the Land of the Living Dead," *Journal of Christian Nursing,* summer 1995, pp. 4-6.

[3]Marsha Niven, "Somebody's Son: A Patient Only a Mother Could Love," *Journal of Christian Nursing,* spring 1995, pp. 28-30.

[4]Joy Sterling, "The American Milk Mama," *Journal of Christian Nursing,* winter 1996, pp. 28-30.

[5]Michael D. Calabria and Janet A. Macrae, *Suggestions for Thought by Florence Nightingale* (Philadelphia: University of Pennsylvania, 1994), p. ix.

[6]Ibid., p. 13.

[7]JoAnn G. Widerquist, "Florence Nightingale's Calling," *Second Opinion,* January 1992, pp. 108-21.

[8]Bonnie Bullough and Vern L. Bullough, "Our Roots: What We Should Know About Nursing's Christian Pioneers," *Journal of Christian Nursing,* winter 1987, p. 12.

[9]Anne H. Bishop and John R. Scudder, "Nursing As a Practice Rather Than an Art or Science," *Nursing Outlook,* March-April 1997, pp. 82-85.

[10]Patricia Benner, ed., *Interpretive Phenomenology: Embodiment, Caring, and Ethics in Health and Illness* (Thousand Oaks, Calif.: Sage, 1994), p. xvii.

[11]Virginia A. Henderson, *The Nature of Nursing: Reflections After 25 Years* (New York: National League for Nursing Press, 1991), p. 21.

[12]Ibid., pp. 22-23.

[13]Martha E. Rogers, *An Introduction to the Theoretical Basis of Nursing* (Philadelphia: F. A. Davis, 1970), p. 122.

[14]Jean Watson, "Nursing's Caring-Healing Paradigm as Exemplar for Alternative Medicine?" *Alternative Therapies,* July 1995, p. 67.

[15]Rosemarie Rizzo Parse, *Illuminations: The Human Becoming Theory in Practice and Research* (New York: National League for Nursing Press, 1995), p. 82.

[16]These health care providers include midwives, shamans and wise women, but none of these roles meet the criteria for professional nursing as defined in this chapter.

[17]Patricia Donahue, *Nursing: The Finest Art—An Illustrated History* (St. Louis, Mo.: Mosby, 1985), p. 93.

[18]Josephine Dolan, M. Louise Fitzpatrick and Eleanor Krohn Herrmann, *Nursing in Society: A Historical Perspective,* 15th ed. (Philadelphia: W. B. Saunders, 1983), p. 43.

[19]James Monroe Barnett, *The Diaconate: A Full and Equal Order* (Valley Forge, Pa.: Trinity

Press, 1995), pp. 28-42.

[20]David Zersen, "Parish Nursing: 20th-Century Fad?" *Journal of Christian Nursing*, spring 1994, pp. 19-21, 45.

[21]Dolan et al., *Nursing in Society*, p. 45.

[22]Mary Haazig, "Historical Presence of the Nurse in the Church," in *Oneness in Purpose—Diversity in Practice* (Park Ridge, Ill.: National Parish Nurse Resource Center, 1989), p. 3.

[23]Bullough and Bullough, "Our Roots," pp. 11-12.

[24]Lavinia L. Dock and Isabel Maitland Stewart, *A Short History of Nursing, From the Earliest Times to the Present Day* (New York: Putnam, 1931), p. 51.

[25]Verna Benner Carson, *Spiritual Dimensions of Nursing Practice* (Philadelphia: W. B. Saunders, 1989), p. 57.

[26]Ibid., pp. 59-60.

[27]Dock and Stewart, *A Short History of Nursing*, p. 99.

[28]Dolan et al., *Nursing in Society*, p. 137.

[29]Charles Dickens, *Martin Chuzzlewit* (New York: Books, Inc., 1868). Sairey Gamp is introduced in chapter 19 and continues as a key figure for the remainder of the book.

[30]Ibid., pp. 137-39.

[31]Abdel Ross Wentz, *Fliedner the Faithful* (Philadelphia: Board of Publication of the United Lutheran Church in America, 1936), pp. 55-83.

[32]Mary Lewis Coakley, "Florence Nightingale: A One-Woman Revolution," *Journal of Christian Nursing*, winter 1989, pp. 20-25.

[33]William Passavant in C. Golder, *The History of the Deaconess Movement* (Cincinnati: Jennings and Pye, 1903), p. 585.

[34]See, for example, Diane Hamilton, "Constructing the Mind of Nursing," *Nursing History Review* 2 (1994): 3-28; and Dock and Stewart, *A Short History of Nursing*, pp. 241-83.

[35]Dock and Stewart, *A Short History of Nursing*, pp. 256-57.

[36]Hamilton, "Constructing the Mind of Nursing," pp. 21-22.

[37]Charlotte A. Aikens, *Studies in Ethics for Nurses* (Philadelphia: W. A. Saunders, 1924), pp. 51-52.

[38]Rebecca H. McNeill, "The Ideal Nurse," *American Journal of Nursing* 10, no. 3 (1910): 393.

[39]Dock and Stewart, *A Short History of Nursing*, pp. 187-91.

[40]See for example, Lynn Keegan, *The Nurse as Healer* (Albany, N.Y.: Delmar, 1994), pp. 182-88.

[41]Margaret J. Dunlop, in Patricia Benner, *Interpretive Phenomenology* (Thousand Oaks, Calif.: Sage, 1994), p. 31.

[42]Verna Carson, "Caring: The Rediscovery of Our Nursing Roots," *Perspectives in Psychiatric Care*, April-June 1994, pp. 4-6.

[43]American Nurses Association, *Summary of the Lewin-VHI, Inc., Report: Nursing Report Card for Acute Care Settings* (Washington, D.C.: American Nurses Association, 1995).

[44]Susan Stocker, "Pretty Scary Stuff," *The American Nurse*, September 1995, p. 6.

Chapter 2: Revolution in the Nursing Paradigm

[1]The three stories are composites of situations the writers have encountered.

[2]Virginia Henderson, *The Nature of Nursing* (New York: Macmillan, 1966), p. 15. "The unique function of the nurse is to assist the individual, sick or well, in the performance of those activities contributing to health or its recovery (or to peaceful death) that he would perform unaided if he had the necessary strength, will or knowledge. And to do this in such a way as to help him gain independence as rapidly as possible."

[3]See, for example, Hildegard E. Peplau, *Interpersonal Relations in Nursing* (New York: Putnam, 1952); Joyce Travelbee, *Interpersonal Aspects of Nursing* (Philadelphia: F. A. Davis, 1971).

[4]Positivist science is characterized by three features: presuppositionless objectivity, being empirically testable by experiments, and rationality. Bruce R. Reichenbach and V. Elving Anderson, *On Behalf of God: A Christian Ethic for Biology* (Grand Rapids, Mich: Eerdmans, 1995), p. 16.

[5]Thomas S. Kuhn, *The Structure of Scientific Revolutions*, 2nd ed. (Chicago: University of Chicago Press, 1970). Kuhn assumes that nature exists, and it is when the facts of nature no longer seem to fit within the prevailing theories that scientists are pushed to adopt new paradigms, ways of thinking about the part of nature they are studying. "Nature itself must first undermine professional security by making prior achievements seem problematic" (p. 169). However, when scientists are operating on the basis of differing paradigms they see reality differently (p. 150).

[6]Ibid., pp. 170-72.

[7]See the chapter by Sue Marquis Bishop, "History and Philosophy of Science," in *Nursing Theorists and Their Work*, ed. Ann Marriner-Tomey, 3rd ed. (St. Louis, Mo.: Mosby, 1994), pp. 27-36.

[8]Naturalistic theories assume that reality is only empirical, natural. There is no account of God or spirit in these theories.

[9]Martha A. Rogers, *An Introduction to the Theoretical Basis of Nursing* (Philadelphia: F. A. Davis, 1970).

[10]Rogers's book in nursing is comparable to Kuhn's for the larger scientific community in that both formulated a new way to approach the work of their respective disciplines.

[11]Jean Watson, *Human Science and Human Care* (New York: National League for Nursing, 1988); Margaret A. Newman, *Health as Expanding Consciousness*, 2nd ed. (New York: National League for Nursing, 1994).

[12]Barbara J. Stevens Barnum, *Nursing Theory: Analysis, Application, Evaluation*, 4th ed. (Philadelphia: Lippincott, 1994), pp. 251-52.

[13]Ontology is the study of being, of what exists, of ultimate reality. Its investigations concern what exists beyond what is directly observable, and its conclusions are arrived at by logic and speculation. For example, philosophers have constructed ontological arguments for the existence of God. While these have logical value, Christians believe that God has revealed himself in Jesus Christ. In Indo-European ontology, what ultimately exists are the two powers of good and evil. In modern naturalism, matter is what ultimately exists.

[14]Ibid., p. 269.

[15]We think that Kuhn is correct if we operate as he does from a naturalistic understanding of reality. We think that there is a way to bring about conversation. It is based on an understanding that reality is the creation of God and that God has revealed to us a way to think about reality.

[16]June F. Kikuchi and Helen Simmons, eds. *Philosophic Inquiry in Nursing* (Newbury Park, Calif.: Sage, 1992).

[17]"Nursing, as a professional community, must have and hold a common, recitable ideology just as nations have their constitutional preambles and pledges of allegiance, fraternal societies have their oaths, religions have their creed." Margretta Styles, quoted in Luci Young Kelly and Lucille A. Joel, *Dimensions of Professional Nursing*, 7th ed. (New York: McGraw-Hill, 1995), p. 208.

[18]Paul G. Hiebert, *Anthropological Reflections on Missiological Issues* (Grand Rapids, Mich.: Baker, 1994), pp. 11-12.

[19]Ibid., p. 36.

[20]Ibid., p. 204.

[21]Ibid., pp. 204-5.

[22]The term *dualism* is used in several different ways. In philosophy *metaphysical dualism* is the view that reality consists of two irreducible principles or entities of opposition that can never be reconciled. In theology it is the idea that the world is ruled by antagonistic forces of good and evil, or that human beings have two basic natures, the physical and the spiritual. Other dualism are between mind and matter, chance and necessity, will and intellect, natural and supernatural, and positive and negative. Dualism carries the implication that the two entities are so radically different that no communication or agreement is possible between them. Eternal struggle for mastery exists between these two entities.

Some writers differentiate between the hard dualism described above and a soft dualism. This softer dualism recognizes distinctions without claiming that they are necessarily opposed and acknowledges that they may influence each other. We prefer the word *distinction* instead of soft dualism.

Nurses who espouse holistic theories want to overcome hard dualism. For example, Rogers rejected earlier definitions of person as biophysical, psychosocial and spiritual beings, preferring the idea of persons as irreducible, indivisible wholes.

[23]Bruce R. Reichenbach and V. Elving Anderson, *On Behalf of God: A Christian Ethic for Biology* (Grand Rapids, Mich.: Eerdmans, 1995), p. 11. English philosopher Francis Bacon (1561-1626) called himself the "trumpeter of his times." He sought to reform science, which until then had been influenced by Aristotle's search for essences. He advocated empirical science instead. "For Bacon, the function of science ultimately was to control nature for human benefit." He believed that science was a form of power. To exercise power over nature we must understand nature and its causes or principles.

[24]Consider, for example, the constitution of United States in which life, liberty and the pursuit of happiness are the purpose of human life. The founders of America were strongly influenced by Enlightenment thinking.

[25]Hiebert, *Anthropological Reflections*, p. 221.

[26]For those who want to read more about the development called postmodernism, we

recommend the following: Albert Borgmann, *Crossing the Postmodern Divide* (Chicago: University of Chicago Press, 1992); Stanley J. Grenz, *A Primer on Postmodernism* (Grand Rapids, Mich.: Eerdmans, 1996); Dennis McCallum, ed., *The Death of Truth* (Minneapolis: Bethany House, 1996); Pauline Marie Rosenau, *Post-Modernism and the Social Sciences* (Princeton, N.J.: Princeton University Press, 1992); Gene Edward Veith, *Postmodern Times: A Christian Guide to Contemporary Thought and Culture* (Wheaton, Ill.: Crossway, 1994); Nicholas Wolterstorff, "Does Truth Still Matter? Reflections on the Crisis of the Postmodern University," *CRUX,* September 1995, pp. 17-28.

[27]Dora Kunz and Erik Peper, "Fields and Their Clinical Implications," in *Spiritual Aspects of the Healing Arts,* ed. Dora Kunz (Wheaton, Ill.: Theosophical Publishing House, 1985), pp. 213-61. Also see Rochelle B. Mackey, "Discover the Healing Power of Therapeutic Touch," *American Journal of Nursing,* April 1995, pp. 27-31.

[28]Barbara Blattner, *Holistic Nursing* (Englewood Cliffs, N.J.: Prentice-Hall, 1981), pp. 7-16; and Lynn Keegan, *The Nurse as Healer* (Albany, N.Y.: Delmar, 1994), pp. 4-6.

[29]Sharon Fish, "Therapeutic Touch: Can We Trust the Data?" *Journal of Christian Nursing,* summer 1993, pp. 6-7.

[30]One of the most-quoted is Fritjof Capra, *The Tao of Physics* (Boulder, Colo.: Shambhala, 1975).

[31]Nobel Prize-winning physicist Leon Lederman, *The God Particle* (New York: Bantam Doubleday Dell, 1993), provides an entertaining exposé in his chapter "The Dancing Moo-Shu Masters," pp. 189-98.

[32]Hiebert, *Anthropological Reflections,* p. 196.

[33]Ibid., p. 224.

[34]Sharon Fish, "Therapeutic Touch: Healing Science or Metaphysical Fraud?" and "A Brief History of Theosophy," *Journal of Christian Nursing,* summer 1996, pp. 4-13.

[35]Hiebert, *Anthropological Reflections,* p. 224.

[36]Mircea Eliade, *Shamanism: Archaic Techniques of Ecstasy,* trans. W. R. Trask (Princeton, N.J.: Princeton University Press, 1972), pp. 3-8.

[37]An example is the work by Jeanne Achterberg, who teaches and is involved in rehabilitation research at the University of Texas Health Science Center in Dallas. Her 1985 book *Imagery in Healing: Shamanism and Modern Medicine* is often cited in reference lists of nurses who write about holistic health. In this book she attempts to explain the power of shamans to heal by the science of psychoneuroimmunology. In her 1994 *Rituals of Healing,* written with nurses Barbara Dossey and Leslie Kolkmeier, she refers to crosscultural studies of shamanic and other rituals that have led to her conclusions. In February 1996 Dr. Larry Dossey appeared on the TV program *Unsolved Mysteries,* supporting the use of shamanistic practices in modern health care.

[38]In May 1993 one of the authors, Arlene, attended a workshop at Harrisburg Area Community College taught by Janet Quinn, well-known teacher of Therapeutic Touch. Dr. Quinn said that the hand movements of TT were for the benefit of the healer and that eventually could be dispensed with. The clear implication was that healing would occur by mental concentration only.

[39]One writer interprets James 5:13-17 as affirming the innate power of people to heal. Tom

Countryman, "Energy-Based Healing Arts and Christian Teaching," *Beginnings: The Official Newsletter of the American Holistic Nurses Association,* January 1996, p. 9. He fails to say that it is the Lord who will raise up the sick. To pray in the name of the Lord is to use delegated authority and to attribute the power to God, not to the healer. He also omits the references to confession and forgiveness of sin as part of healing. Only God can forgive sin.

[40]Historian Eugene D. Dukes traces the history of the attitude of the Christian church toward the practice of magic. He notes that the distinction between white magic *(theurgia)* and black magic *(goeteia)* was made by the Greeks and Romans. "Generally speaking, while the practice of the former in Greece and Rome was considered beneficial to society, the latter inspired fear and provoked condemnation." *Magic and Witchcraft in the Dark Ages* (Lanham, Md.: University Press of America, 1995), p. 53.

[41]Ibid. Scholars regard witchcraft as the social dimension of magic.

[42]Shirley H. Fondiller and Barbara J. Nerone, *Nursing: the Career of a Lifetime* (New York: National League for Nursing Press, 1995). This book is written for men and women either just entering or considering nursing.

[43]In 1994 one of the continuing education offerings at the American Nurses Association Convention was on witchery and crones. References to the triple goddess appear in some of the nursing literature. Spencer et al. (see note 44 below) write that modern-day witches claim to be priestesses of the ancient European shamanistic nature religion that worships a goddess related to the ancient Mother Goddess in her three aspects of maiden, mother and crone. p. 25.

[44]Aïda Besançon Spencer with Donna F. G. Hailson, Catherine Clark Kroeger, and William David Spencer, *The Goddess Revival* (Grand Rapids, Mich.: Baker, 1995), pp. 202-3. The authors have carefully documented their conclusions from historical, contemporary and biblical research. They offer practical suggestions for those wanting to leave the practice of Wicca.

Chapter 3: A Biblical Worldview for Nursing

[1]Ingeborg Gjersvik, "A Heart of Compassion: How Nursing Started in Norway," *Journal of Christian Nursing,* spring 1997, p. 12.

[2]Eusebius of Caesarea, as quoted in Josephine Dolan, M. Louise Fitzpatrick and Eleanor Krohn Herrmann, *Nursing in Society: A Historical Perspective,* 15th ed. (Philadelphia: W. B. Saunders, 1983), p. 43.

[3]Ibid.

[4]Timothy F. Lull, *Called to Confess Christ* (Philadelphia: Parish Life, 1980), p. 37.

[5]See Isaiah 44 for a graphic description of how God views our idolatry.

[6]Ann Bradshaw, *Lighting the Lamp: the Spiritual Dimension of Nursing Care* (London: Scutari, 1994), pp. 97-169.

[7]A word picture from the Old Testament envisions people being "bound in the bundle of the living under the care of the Lord your God" (1 Sam 25:29). Another picture is that of being held in God's hand: "In his hand is the life of every living thing and the breath of every human being" (Job 12:10). God is seen as a life-giving fountain of water: "For with you is the fountain of life; in your light we see light" (Ps 36:9). God is like a protective trail

guide: "Bless our God, O peoples, let the sound of his praise be heard, who has kept us among the living, and has not let our feet slip" (Ps 66:9).

[8]Martin Luther, *Luther's Small Catechism*, trans. Timothy Wengert (Minneapolis: Augsburg Fortress, 1996, original 1536), p. 21.

[9]Carl R. Rogers, *On Becoming a Person* (Boston: Houghton Mifflin, 1961), p. 26. Rogers asserts that this understanding of persons as having strongly positive directional tendencies was basic to his personality theory.

[10]Jacqueline Fawcett, *Analysis and Evaluation of Conceptual Models of Nursing*, 3rd ed. (Philadelphia: F. A. Davis, 1995), p. 7.

[11]Ibid.

[12]Margaret A. Newman, *Health as Expanding Consciousness* (St. Louis: Mosby-Year Book, 1987).

[13]Rosemarie Risso Parse, "Human Becoming: Parse's Theory of Nursing," *Nursing Science Quarterly*, 5 (1992): 35-42.

Chapter 4: What Does It Mean to Be Human?

[1]Roberta M. Gilbert, *Extraordinary Relationships: A New Way of Thinking About Human Interactions* (Minneapolis: Chronimed, 1992), p. viii. Despite Bowen's apparent dislike for the doctrine of the *imago Dei*, his theory is actually quite compatible with Christian thought.

[2]Dorothy Kleffel, *Exploring Our Environmental Connections* (New York: National League for Nursing Press, 1994), p. 9.

[3]Paul K. Jewett, *Who We Are: Our Dignity as Human* (Grand Rapids, Mich.: Eerdmans, 1996), p. 23.

[4]Jürgen Moltmann, *Man: Christian Anthropology in the Conflicts of the Present* (Philadelphia: Fortress Press, 1974), p. 20.

[5]Em Olivia Bevis, *Curriculum Building in Nursing: A Process* (New York: National League for Nursing Press, 1989), pp. 43-44.

[6]Consider, for example, Abraham, who twice allowed his wife to be taken into a foreign king's harem because he feared for his own life (Gen 12; 20). Lot offered his virgin daughters to an angry local mob to be raped (Gen 19). Jacob deceived his brother out of his birthright to become a patriarch of the nation of Israel (Gen 27).

[7]See, for example, Isaiah 1:17; Psalm 82:3; Job 31:18-22; Jeremiah 7:5-6; Ezekiel 22:7; Zechariah 7:9-10.

[8]Hans Walter Wolff, *Anthropology of the Old Testament* (Philadelphia: Fortress, 1974), p. 8.

[9]For example, Isaiah 52:7, "How beautiful upon the mountains are the feet of him who brings good tidings," refers not to the appearance of the feet but to their function in bringing the message.

[10]Here *Greek* refers to the Greek language, not Greek philosophy.

[11]Rudolf Bultmann, *Theology of the New Testament* (New York: Scribner's, 1951), p. 205.

[12]Ibid., pp. 220-21.

[13]Raymond E. Brown, Joseph A. Fitzmyer and Roland E. Murphy, *The Jerome Biblical*

Commentary (Englewood Cliffs, N.J.: Prentice-Hall, 1968), p. 820.

[14]Jewett, *Who We Are*, p. 38.

[15]1 Cor 6:19. The temple was viewed as the dwelling place of God by the Jewish people. In Christianity this was expanded to realizing that God dwelt among and within his people.

[16]For two helpful resources see Tim Stafford, *The Sexual Christian* (Wheaton, Ill.: Victor, 1989); and Lewis B. Smedes, *Sex for Christians: The Limits and Liberties of Sexual Living* (Grand Rapids, Mich.: Eerdmans, 1994).

[17]Bernard J. Klamecki, in *The Crisis of Homosexuality*, ed. J. Isamu Yamamoto (Wheaton, Ill.: Victor, 1990), p. 119.

[18]Lawlessness—which was the charge that Martin Luther faced from his critics when he insisted that we are saved by grace alone.

Chapter 5: The Person as a Spiritual Being

[1]Dallas Willard, *The Spirit of the Disciplines* (San Francisco: Harper SanFrancisco, 1988), p. 77.

[2]Ibid., p. 78.

[3]Joan E. Haase, Teri Britt, Doris D. Coward, Nancy Kline Leidy and Patricia E. Penn, "Simultaneous Concept Analysis of Spiritual Perspective, Hope, Acceptance and Self-transcendence," *Image*, summer 1992, p. 143.

[4]Ibid.

[5]Julia D. Emblen, "*Religion* and *Spirituality* Defined According to Current Use in Nursing Literature," *Journal of Professional Nursing*, January-February 1992, p. 41.

[6]Margaret A. Burkhardt, "Spirituality: An Analysis of the Concept," *Holistic Nursing Practice*, April 1989, p. 71.

[7]Ibid., pp. 73-74.

[8]Dallas Willard, "What Makes Spirituality Christian?" *Christianity Today*, March 6 995, p. 16.

[9]Steve Turner, "Lean, Green & Meaningless," *Christianity Today*, September 24, 1990, pp. 26-27.

[10]Ibid.

[11]Gerhard O. Forde, "A Lutheran Response," in *Christian Spirituality*, ed. Donald L. Alexander (Downers Grove, Ill.: InterVarsity Press, 1988), p. 192.

[12]Elizabeth L. Hillstrom, *Testing the Spirits* (Downers Grove, Ill.: InterVarsity Press, 1995), p. 132.

[13]Richard J. Foster, *Prayer: Finding the Heart's True Home* (San Francisco: HarperSanFrancisco, 1992), p. 149.

[14]George A. Lane, *Christian Spirituality—An Historical Sketch* (Chicago: Loyola University Press, 1984), p. 2.

[15]E. M. Yamauchi, "Gnosticism," in *New Dictionary of Theology*, ed. Sinclair B. Ferguson, David F. Wright and J. I. Packer (Downers Grove, Ill.: InterVarsity Press, 1988), p. 272.

[16]Robert Brow, *Religion: Origins and Ideas* (Chicago: InterVarsity Press, 1966), pp. 33-36.

[17]Irving Hexham, *Concise Dictionary of Religion* (Downers Grove, Ill.: InterVarsity Press, 1993), p. 153.

[18]Henry Chadwick, *The Early Church* (Grand Rapids, Mich.: Eerdmans, 1967), p. 52.

[19]Linda E. Sabin, "Hildegard of Bingen: A Woman of Vision," *Journal of Christian Nursing,* spring 1997, pp. 8-9.

[20]Lane, *Christian Spirituality,* p. 34.

[21]Monica Furlong, *The Wisdom of Julian of Norwich* (Grand Rapids, Mich.: Eerdmans, 1996), p. 7.

[22]Teresa of Ávila, *Interior Castle,* ed. and trans. E. Allison Peers (New York: Doubleday, 1989), p. 235. The original version of this book was written in 1588.

[23]Liberal Christianity taught this with good biblical reasons! See, for example, Luke 10:25-37; Ephesians 2:10; James 1:26-27; 2:14-26.

[24]Believing the right doctrines, while important, has less biblical precedent. See, for example, Matthew 23:2-3; James 2:19.

[25]Hans Walter Wolff, *Anthropology of the Old Testament* (Philadelphia: Fortress, 1974), pp. 32-39.

[26]Ibid., p. 39.

[27]J. D. G. Dunn, "Spirit, Holy Spirit," in *New Bible Dictionary,* ed. I. Howard Marshall, A. R. Millard, J. I. Packer, and D. J. Wiseman, 3rd ed. (Downers Grove, Ill.: InterVarsity Press, 1996), p. 1125.

Chapter 6: The Person as a Cultural Being

[1]For example, I (Arlene) taught nursing for three years in Zambia. Living in that Bantu culture enriched my understanding of the Bible. The Tonga people, among whom I lived, understood the power of anger in a way that deepened my appreciation for Paul's injunction: "Be angry but do not sin; do not let the sun go down on your anger, and do not make room for the devil" (Eph 4:26-27). Anger was the precursor to cursing and all sorts of evil for the Tonga. This illustrated Paul's warning that nursing anger was making room for the devil.

[2]Madeleine M. Leininger, ed., *Culture Care Diversity and Universality: A Theory of Nursing* (New York: National League for Nursing Press, 1991).

[3]Rachel E. Spector, *Cultural Diversity in Health and Illness,* 4th ed. (Stamford, Conn.: Appleton & Lange, 1996). Dr. Spector's book includes many listings of resources for those interested in further information about cultural health practices.

[4]Charles Sherlock, *The Doctrine of Humanity* (Downers Grove, Ill.: InterVarsity Press, 1996), p. 131.

[5]Ibid.

[6]S. D. Gaede, *When Tolerance Is No Virtue* (Downers Grove, Ill.: InterVarsity Press, 1993).

[7]Bruce J. Nicholls, *Contextualization: A Theology of Gospel and Culture* (Downers Grove, Ill.: InterVarsity Press, 1979), pp. 11-12.

[8]This model is suggested by G. Linwood Barney and is discussed in Nicholls, *Contextualization,* p. 11.

[9]These seven worldview questions are the model proposed by James W. Sire in *The Universe Next Door,* 3rd ed. (Downers Grove, Ill.: InterVarsity Press, 1997), pp. 17-18. There are other models, but we have found this one helpful. It has guided much of our thinking for this book.

[10]Nicholls, *Contextualization*, p. 13.

[11]Ibid.

[12]Church history attests to the influence of culture on the beliefs and practices of Christians; hence the need for prophetic voices and constant reformation.

[13]See chapter four.

[14]Eugene D. Dukes, *Magic and Witchcraft in the Dark Ages* (Lanham, Md.: University Press of America, 1996), p. 266.

[15]Barry G. Webb, *The Message of Isaiah* (Downers Grove, Ill.: InterVarsity Press, 1996), p. 180.

[16]Ibid., p. 181.

[17]Ibid., p. 180.

[18]"The World Evangelical Fellowship Manila Declaration," in *The Unique Christ In Our Pluralist World*, ed. Bruce J. Nicholls (Grand Rapids, Mich.: Baker, 1994), p. 16.

[19]Spector, *Cultural Diversity*, pp. 14-16.

[20]Barbara Montgomery Dossey says that the concept of *transpersonal self* (a self-induced movement toward greater health—physical, mental, emotional, spiritual) is based on the Patanjali system of yoga, as well as theosophy, Buddhism, Hinduism, Sufism and American Indian philosophy. "Transpersonal Self and States of Consciousness," in *Holistic Health Promotion: A Guide for Practice*, ed. Barbara Montgomery Dossey, Lynn Keegan, Leslie Goodling Kolkmeier and Cathie E. Guzzetta (Rockville, Md.: Aspen, 1999), p. 30.

Larry Dossey asserts that three principles underlie prayer: (1) there is a telepathic link between all people, plants, stones, and heaven and earth; (2) the universe is a pulsating unity to which anyone can open themselves; and (3) empathic attunement with all things. These principles can be used for good or ill and are the same principles on which shamanism and hexing operate. These principles "operate at deep levels, whether we know it or not." Larry Dossey, *Healing Words* (San Francisco: HarperSanFrancisco, 1993), p. 150. These principles are the essence of spiritual monism, the belief that there are no distinctions in reality.

Deepak Chopra quotes freely from Hindu, Taoist and Buddhist texts to support his claims that aging can be prevented by right thinking in *Ageless Body, Timeless Mind: The Quantum Alternative to Growing Old* (New York: Harmony Books, 1993).

Andrew Weil advocates the Zen Buddhist form of meditation in *Natural Health, Natural Medicine* (Boston: Houghton Mifflin, 1995), p. 126. Each of these authors are not believers in the sense that they would identify themselves with any one of these religions. They are much more pragmatic. Only if these techniques work for the individual are they considered helpful.

[21]WEF Manila Declaration, in *Unique Christ in Our Pluralist World*, p. 15.

[22]Even C. Everett Koop, who openly professes his Christian faith, seems to approve of this pragmatic approach to health. He writes in a medical textbook of complementary medicine: "My experience with physicians has convinced me that they are healers first. As such, they are willing to use any ethical approach or treatment that has been proven to work." To his credit, he does call for scientific research to assess the usefulness of alternative medicine. Nevertheless, the criterion is still usefulness. C. Everett Koop, foreword to *Fundamentals of Complementary and Alternative Medicine*, ed. Marc S. Micozzi (New York:

Churchill Livingstone, 1995), p. xi.

[23]Jeanne Achterberg, Barbara Dossey and Leslie Kolkmeier, *Rituals of Healing* (New York: Bantam, 1994) p. 4.

[24]Conversation with Sharon Fish, who interviewed practitioners of therapeutic touch. One practitioner became a spirit medium after several years of involvement in therapeutic touch.

[25]We have found that many Christian nurses are unable to discern the difference between a biblical understanding of reality and those of other faiths. As a result, guided by good intentions to be helpful but also by the cultural virtue of tolerance, they naively adopt practices that are antithetical to saying, "Jesus is Lord." Sometimes this error stems from lack of knowledge; however, it also come from an inability to view all of life, including nursing, from a biblical perspective.

[26]An example is Chinese medicine. The benefit of various herbs and other substances are explained by the *yin* and *yang*, the two energies that must be in harmonious relationship for health. Indeed, many of these substances may be beneficial physiologically, and research is being conducted to isolate the active ingredients.

[27]June F. Kikuchi, Helen Simmons and Donna Romyn, eds., *Truth in Nursing Inquiry* (Thousand Oaks, Calif.: Sage, 1996), pp. 151-54.

[28]Charles Sherlock, *The Doctrine of Humanity* (Downers Grove, Ill.: InterVarsity Press, 1996), pp. 135-37. "Customs such as human sacrifice, female circumcision, widow-burning, foot-binding, prostitution, slavery and torture are clearly opposed to God's will for human life. Others are less obviously wrong, but reinforce sinful attitudes such as selfishness, greed or lust; television commercials provide plenty of evidence in the highly ambiguous culture of consumerism. Even in those aspects of a culture which embody the highest ideals to which human beings aspire, or which celebrate the goodness of God that pervades everyday life, sin is present. Consider birth, retirement, setting up a new home, or beginning a meal: a child can be seen only as evidence of a parent's achievement, whether in fertility or child-rearing; retirement as boasting or escaping to laziness; a new home can provide the chance for ostentatious display; and even grace at the table can be a means of controlling behavior. Indeed the worst idols are precisely the best things set in the place of God, and it is their God-given goodness which makes them attractive" (pp. 137-38).

Chapter 7: The Seen Environment

[1]Diane Garey and Lawrence R. Hott, *Sentimental Women Need Not Apply: A History of the American Nurse.* VHS format. Florentine Films/L. Hatt and D. Garey, 1988.

[2]"In watching diseases, both in private homes and in public hospitals, the things which strikes the experienced observer most forcibly is this, that the symptoms or the sufferings generally considered to be inevitable and incident to the disease are very often not symptoms of the disease at all, but of something quite different—of the want of fresh air, or of light, or of warmth, or of quiet, or of cleanliness, or of punctuality and care in the administration of diet, or each or all of these." Florence Nightingale, *Notes on Nursing: What It Is and What It Is Not* (1860; reprint, New York: Appleton, Dover, 1969), p. 8.

[3]Committee on Enhancing Environmental Health Content in Nursing Practice. The

committee was established by the Institute of Medicine and published its report: Andrew M. Pope, Meta A. Snyder and Lillian H. Mood, eds., *Nursing, Health, & the Environment: Strengthening the Relationship to Improve the Public's Health* (Washington, D.C.: National Academy Press, 1995).

[4]Dorothy Kleffel, "The Environment: Alive, Whole and Interacting," in *Exploring Our Environmental Connections,* ed. Eleanor A. Schuster and Carolyn Brown (New York: National League for Nursing Press, 1994), pp. 14-15.

[5]Ibid.

[6]George Howe Colt, "See Me, Feel Me, Touch Me, Heal Me," *Life,* August 1996, pp.34-50.

[7]Kleffel, "Environment," p. 7.

[8]Ibid., p. 12.

[9]Jean Watson, "Myth, Mystery, and Metaphors for Ecocaring," in ibid., p. 35.

[10]Martha E. Rogers, *An Introduction to the Theoretical Basis of Nursing* (Philadelphia: F. A. Davis, 1970), p. 118. Martha Rogers first opened the door for nursing to think more expansively of the human environment. She asks, "Can human field boundaries be identified within the space-time dimensions?" While Rogers stresses the mutual interaction and modification of persons and the environment, she is also optimistic about the positive direction of evolutionary change in both. Conscious human interventions for changing both themselves and the environment merely assist in this positive movement.

[11]Joseph E. Pissorno Jr., "Naturopathic Medicine," in *Fundamentals of Complementary and Alternative Medicine,* ed. Marc S. Micozzi (New York: Churchill Livingstone, 1955), pp. 170-73.

[12]Edward B. Davis and Michael Hunter write the following about the scientific revolution of the seventeenth century: "Perhaps most fundamental, however, was the adoption at this time of a new world view, involving a complete change in the way in which nature was conceived. . . . The mechanical philosophers of the seventeenth century challenged prevailing Aristotelian and Galenic notions, which typically depicted nature as a wise and benevolent being. Associated with such views were phrases like 'Nature does nothing in vain,' 'Nature abhors a vacuum' and 'Nature is the wisest physician.' By contrast, thinkers such as René Descartes (1596-1650), Pierre Gassendi (1592-1655) and Robert Boyle (1627-91) held that the world was a vast, impersonal machine, incapable of acting consciously." Robert Boyle, in *A Free Enquiry into the Vulgarly Received Notion of Nature,* ed. Edward B. Davis and Michael Hunter (Cambridge: Cambridge University Press, 1966), p. ix.

[13]Robert Boyle (of Boyle's Laws) was a Christian believer as well a scientist. "For Boyle it was inappropriate both scientifically and theologically to speak of 'Nature' doing anything at all. . . . By denying 'Nature' any wisdom of its own, the mechanical conception of nature located purpose where Boyle believed it belonged: over and behind nature, in the mind of a personal God, rather than an impersonal semi-deity, immanent within the world. Ibid., p. x.

[14]This diagnosis was added by the North American Nursing Diagnosis Association in 1994. Lynda Carpenito includes the following notation: "This new addition to the NANDA list is unique for two reasons. It represents a specific theory—human energy field theory—and the interventions utilized require specialized instruction and supervised practice." Lynda

Juall Carpenito, *Nursing Diagnosis,* 6th ed. (Philadelphia: Lippincott, 1995) pp. 355-59.

[15]Physicist Fritjof Capra popularized the parallels (in his view) between recent developments in physics and Eastern mysticism. In the preface to the first edition (1976) of his book *The Tao of Physics,* he explains how repeated mystical meditative experiences helped him to realize the consistency between modern physics and Eastern mysticism. By 1984 he would write in the revised edition that widespread reception of the book had confirmed his feeling that what he wrote would become common knowledge. He writes, "The philosophy of mystical traditions, also known as the 'perennial philosophy,' provide the most consistent philosophical background to our modern scientific theories" (*The Tao of Physics,* rev. ed. [New York: Bantam, 1984] p. xviii).

[16]" 'Mechanics' is the study of motion, and quantum mechanics refers to the study of the motion of entities that are small enough and move fast enough to have both observable wavelike and particle-like properties. When quantum mechanics is applied to large-scale, familiar phenomena, the effects are too small to be significant and we are left with the laws of classical mechanics intact. Classical mechanics and quantum mechanics are in a sense at the opposite ends of the same continuum" (Therald Moeller, John C. Bailar Jr., Jacob Kleinberg, Cyrus O. Guss, Mary E. Castellion and Clyde Metz, eds., *Chemistry with Inorganic Qualitative Analysis,* 2nd ed. (San Diego, Calif.: Harcourt Brace Jovanovich, 1984), p. 208.

The Heisenberg Uncertainty Principle states, "It is impossible to know simultaneously both the exact momentum and the exact position of an electron." This principle is significant only at the subatomic level. But some view this principle as an intrinsic property of nature, some as a statement of the limits of our knowledge, and others as a matter for philosophical thought.

[17]"He (Bohm) sees mind and matter as being interdependent and correlated, but not causally connected. They are mutually enfolding projections of a higher reality which is neither matter nor consciousness" (Capra, *The Tao of Physics,* p. 310).

[18]Hari M. Sharma, "Maharishi Ayruveda," in ed., *Fundamentals of Complementary and Alternative Medicine,* pp. 243-54.

[19]There has been a strong belief in the West that physics and chemistry alone could not explain life. Carl Sagan discusses the postulation of a *vital force,* an *entelechy,* a *tau* or a *mana* the animated life. Eighteenth-century chemist Joseph Priestly tried to find the *vital force* by weighing a mouse just before and just after it died. Of course it weighed the same. Sagan quips, "If there is soul-stuff, evidently it weighs nothing—that is it is not made of matter." *The Demon Haunted World: Science as a Candle in the Dark* (New York: Random House, 1995), p. 272.

[20]"The biosphere is a symphony of symphonies. The creatures that inhabit earth's ecosystems maintain and sustain the living fabric of the biosphere—as they reproduce, they continue to bring forth life from death. Through all this process they cycle and recycle the basic stuff of creation, all powered by the sun. And over all this activity, God provides everything these creatures need to continue through the years and generations." Calvin B. DeWitt, *Earthwise* (Grand Rapids, Mich.: CRC Publications, 1994), p. 19.

[21]"This is an expression of God's judgment, and indication of coming misfortune. The blessings are reversed. The joyous dance of creation becomes a dirge, as a shadow falls over things" (David Atkinson, *The Message of Genesis 1—11* (Downers Grove, Ill.: InterVarsity Press, 1990), p. 93.

[22]Fred Van Dyke, David C. Mahan, Joseph K. Sheldon and Raymond H. Brand, *Redeeming Creation: The Biblical Basis for Environmental Stewardship* (Downers Grove, Ill.: InterVarsity Press, 1996), p. 91.

[23]Ibid., pp. 163-64.

[24]The classification is developed by P. Stevens and J. Hall in 1993. It was reprinted in Andrew M. Pope, Meta A. Snyder and Lillian H. Mood, eds., *Nursing, Health, & the Environment* (Washington, D.C.: National Academy Press, 1995), pp. 27-28.

[25]Sherwin Nuland writes about the fascination of physicians with solving the puzzle of an illness in his book *How We Die* (New York: Alfred A. Knopf, 1994).

Chapter 8: The Unseen Environment

[1]I (Arlene) was in a masters program in a school of public health from 1968-1970. During those years Federal money was pouring into programs developed in response to President Lyndon Johnson's 1964 "War on Poverty." Many of these programs were good ones, at least in theory, like Head Start Programs and community based mental health clinics, etc. Many individuals benefited from them. But the hoped for lifting of entire social groups out of poverty did not work out. Today, we read much about the increasing disparity between the growing poor underclass in the United States and those who are becoming increasingly wealthy.

[2]Anthropologist Kristofer Schipper writes out of his own study of and involvement with Taoism. The highest goal of this ancient belief and practice is "Long Life." On the surface there appears to be little left of Taoism, but Schipper sees its presence in the revival of health and longevity practices of *qigong* and Chinese medicine. Kristofer Schipper, *The Taoist Body* (Berkeley: University of California Press, 1993), p. 9.

[3]David Mains and Karen Mains, *Tales of the Kingdom* (Elgin, Ill.: David C. Cook, 1983).

[4]Donald G. Bloesch, *Jesus Christ: Savior & Lord* (Downers Grove, Ill.: InterVarsity Press, 1997), p. 237.

[5]Paul tells us to test the spirits and not to accept all claims of spiritual insight as truth (1 Thess 5:19-21). The Bible warns repeatedly about false prophets and miracles (Mk 13:22; Deut 13: 1-5). We are told to judge all such claims *theologically*—how they agree with the rest of what we know about God as found in Scripture—and *morally*—how the lives of those claiming such insight and knowledge are evidence of godly living. The ultimate test is whether or not the person recognizes Jesus Christ as Savior and Lord.

[6]Donald G. Bloesch, *Holy Scripture: Revelation, Inspiration & Interpretation* (Downers Grove, Ill.: InterVarsity Press, 1994), p. 53.

[7]Bloesch, *Jesus Christ*, p. 238.

[8]Bloesch, *Holy Scripture*, p. 48.

[9]Many religions see the struggle between good an evil as an eternal one; first one prevails

and then the other. The Scriptures give us no such picture. Rather, the story of the Bible is how God works throughout history to bring those who so desire into his kingdom. Finally, the two kingdoms will no longer exist together and God's kingdom will prevail. See Revelation 11:15, 17.

[10]St. Paul identifies the devil, referred to a Satan in other places, as the ruler of this world. See Ephesians 2:1-2; 6:11-12.

[11]Satan is referred to as a heavenly being who both went about in the earth and was present before the Lord in Job 1:6-8. Jesus referred to Satan as having fallen from heaven in Luke 10:18. Jesus did not dispute the idea that Satan was the ruler of demons in Matthew 12:24-27. The Scriptures are veiled as to the origin of these evil beings while they accept their reality. Many biblical scholars believe that when Satan fell from heaven he took with him a large contingent of angels and that these fallen angels are demons. We think it wise to not say any more than what can be substantiated by Scripture.

[12]Bloesch, *Jesus Christ*, p. 44.

[13]Scripture is clear that we are born prisoners of Satan and that only through Christ can we be rescued from this dark kingdom. When people declare their autonomy they are only fooling themselves. We are actually slaves of sin. "But thanks be to God that you, having once been slaves of sin, have become obedient from the heart to the form of teaching to which you were entrusted" (Rom 6:17).

[14]James Montgomery Boice, *Two Cities, Two Loves* (Downers Grove, Ill.: InterVarsity Press, 1996), pp. 73-75.

[15]Ibid., p. 74.

[16]Ibid., p. 76.

[17]"More than one manager has told me that he loved office politics—the intrigue, the maneuvering—and that he was good at it. These managers manipulated others, tried to divide and conquer staff members, hinted that certain people were not as good at their jobs as others thought, whispered promises they never intended to keep." (p. 20). Cheryl Forbes, *The Religion of Power* (Grand Rapids, Mich.: Zondervan), 1983.

[18]Historian Christopher Lasch, in his extensive writing, exposed the development and collapse of the idea of progress. One example is *The True and Only Heaven* (New York: W. W. Norton, 1991).

[19]The Scripture does characterize sin as disease in some places, but it is a disease brought on by rebellion (Is 1:4-6).

[20]Eugene Peterson, "Teach Us to Care and Not to Care," in *The Crisis of Care*, ed. Susan S. Phillips and Patricia Benner (Washington, D.C.: Georgetown University Press, 1994), p. 70. Eugene Peterson reminds Christians that they of all people should not be naive or ignorant about sin. The Bible is both insistent and convincing on the subject. However, even unbelievers should not have difficulty acknowledging the reality of sin. "It is, as Chesterton once pointed out, the only major Christian doctrine that can be verified empirically."

[21]Judith Allen Shelly and Arlene B. Miller, *Values in Conflict* (Downers Grove, Ill.: InterVarsity Press, 1991), p. 81.

[22]David Atkinson, *The Message of Proverbs* (Downers Grove, Ill.: InterVarsity Press, 1996), p. 57.

[23]John F. Kilner, *Life on the Line: Ethics, Aging, Ending Patients' Lives & Allocating Vital Resources* (Grand Rapids, Mich.: Eerdmans, 1992).

[24]Derek Kidner, as quoted by David Atkinson, *The Message of Genesis 1—11* (Downers Grove, Ill.: InterVarsity Press, 1990), p. 170.

[25]Peterson, "Teach Us to Care," pp. 74-75.

[26]Ibid., p. 73.

Chapter 9: A Storied Environment

[1]Elaine Creasman, "The Patient in Room 321," *Journal of Christian Nursing,* fall 1994, pp. 22-23.

[2]Linda E. Sabin, "Claiming Our Heritage: Bridge to a Lasting Future," *Journal of Christian Nursing,* spring 1997, p. 5.

[3]See chapter one in this book. "Since late antiquity, when Eastern Orthodox Christians established the first hospitals, religious organizations have frequently led the way in providing for the institutional care of the sick." Ronald L. Numbers and Darrel W. Amundsen, eds., *Caring and Curing: Health and Medicine in the Western Religious Traditions* (New York: Macmillan, 1986), p. 2.

[4]Mary Thompson, "Nurturing Hope: A Vital Ingredient in Nursing." *Journal of Christian Nursing,* fall 1994, pp. 10-17.

[5]In their investigation of past research, Carol J. Farran, Kaye A. Herth and Judith M. Popovich conclude, "Although other outcomes may be identified in future qualitative and quantitative studies, there is sufficient evidence to support the biological and psychosocial effects of hope and hopelessness on individuals and families." *Hope and Hopelessness: Critical Clinical Constructs* (Thousand Oaks, Calif.: Sage, 1995), p. 191.

[6]Barbara Sarter, in her study of Martha Rogers's theory, emphasizes that the concept of four-dimensionality (all reality for Rogers) is not space and time. "Reality is nonlinear, nontemporal, nonspatial. . . . nontemporal refers to the relativity of time and to the 'relative present' for a given individual. Paranormal phenomena, such as precognition, telepathy, reincarnation, and meditative modalities, which indicate an awareness 'beyond waking' can be explained by the postulate of four-dimensionality." Barbara Sarter, *The Stream of Becoming* (New York: National League for Nursing, 1988), p. 62. Perhaps the term *timeful* might better express Rogers's meaning. While she rejected the idea of linear time as constraints for people, her ideas of wave phenomena and rhythmicity have no meaning apart from time.

[7]Martha Rogers, *An Introduction to the Theoretical Basis of Nursing* (Philadelphia: F. A. Davis, 1970), pp. 115-16.

[8]Ibid., p. 55. Rogers had a positive view of evolutionary progress. "The theory of progressive evolution finds expression in man's sequential development. The life process is a becoming. The evolution of life exhibits an invariant one-way trend."

[9]Roy Swanstrom, *History in the Making: An Introduction to the Study of the Past* (Downers

Grove, Ill.: InterVarsity Press, 1978), p. 61.

[10]Lillian D. Wald, *Windows on Henry Street* (Boston: Little, Brown, 1934), p. 85.

[11]Ibid., p. 107.

[12]Ibid., p. 336.

[13]We have noted several times that Florence Nightingale's thinking was reflective of this view. Swanstrom observes, "The epitome of the new optimistic spirit was the first world's fair, held in London in 1851, whose huge Crystal Palace attracted thirteen thousand exhibitors and six million visitors and gave dramatic visual demonstrations of human ingenuity and prowess. Without question it left the clear impression that human progress was indeed the key to all history" (*History in the Making,* p. 63). Florence Nightingale would have been thirty years old at this time. The Crimean war, during which she instituted reforms in the care of wounded British soldiers, was fought from 1853-1856. She published *Notes on Nursing,* a book that reflects this positive attitude, in 1860.

[14]Earl B. Erskine, *Hygiene and Public Health* (New York: Prentice-Hall, 1949), p. 4.

[15]Robert W. Jenson, "How the World Lost Its Story," *First Things* 36 (1993): 21.

[16]Mircea Eliade, *The Sacred and the Profane: The Nature of Religion* (New York: Harcourt Brace Jovanovich, 1959), p. 171.

[17]Jenson, "How the World Lost Its Story," p. 21.

[18]I (Arlene) addressed Erikson's theory in my doctoral dissertation, *Becoming Good.* Erikson's well-known chart of developmental stages of the individual ends with the stage of maturity. Some nurse writers refer to death as "the final stage of development," but this seems at best a euphemism. While survivors might be said to "develop" as a result of the death, what about the one who died? The standard response is that answers to this question belong to religion, not nursing. But this is just the point. There is no larger story within which to place our own stories of facing and responding to suffering and death.

[19]"I will be among the few who cheat death of its victory by gaining a reputation that outlives them." David P. Gushee, "How Immortality Almost Killed Me," *Christianity Today,* March 3, 1997, p. 43.

[20]"History," *Holman Bible Dictionary,* CD-ROM edition (Hiawatha, Iowa: Parsons Technology, August 1994).

[21]Scripture tells us that we can seek to know God's ways. Moses, the leader of the Hebrew exodus from Egypt, prayed, "Show me your ways, so that I may know you and find favor in your sight" (Ex 33:13)—a prayer often repeated by God's people since then. This does not mean that God shows us the future; rather, he shows us how to live in such a way that we enter into and cooperate with his plans for us. Because we are made in God's image, our actions have significance "because they contribute to the meaning of the whole."

[22]We are not puppets; we can choose to reject God's purposes (Eph 2:2; Is 65:2).

[23]Eliade, *The Sacred and the Profane,* pp. 111-12.

[24]Phyllis S. Karns, "Building a Foundation for Spiritual Care," *Journal of Christian Nursing,* summer 1991, p. 13.

[25]Susan S. Phillips and Patricia Benner, eds. *The Crisis of Care* (Washington, D.C.: Georgetown University Press, 1994).

[26]Stanley Hauerwas. *The Peaceable Kingdom* (Notre Dame, Ind.: University of Notre Dame Press, 1983), p. 28.

Chapter 10: Working Toward *Shalom*
[1]DeAnn M. Hensley, Kimberly A. Kilgore, Jill Vass Langfitt and LaPhyllis Peterson, "Margaret A. Newman: Model of Health," in *Nursing Theorists and Their Work*, ed. Ann Marriner (St. Louis, Mo.: Mosby, 1986), p. 371.
[2]Rosemarie Risso Parse, "Human Becoming: Parse's Theory of Nursing," *Nursing Science Quarterly* 5 (1992): 13.
[3]Janice B. Lindberg, Mary Love Hunter and Ann Z. Kruszewski, *Introduction to Nursing: Concepts, Issues and Opportunities* (Philadelphia: Lippincott, 1994), pp. 198-99.
[4]Hensley et al., "Margaret A. Newman," p. 371.
[5]Daniel Callahan, "The WHO Definition of 'Health,'" *Hastings Center Studies* 1, no. 3 (1973): 77-87.
[6]Adapted from Judith Allen Shelly and Sharon Fish, *Spiritual Care: the Nurse's Role* (Downers Grove, Illinois: InterVarsity Press, 1988), p. 33.
[7]Madeleine M. Leininger, ed., *Culture Care Diversity and Universality: A Theory of Nursing* (New York: National League for Nursing Press, 1991), p. 6.
[8]Ibid., p. 48.
[9]Bruce J. Malina and Richard L. Rohrbaugh, *Social-Science Commentary on the Synoptic Gospels* (Minneapolis: Fortress, 1992), pp. 70-72.
[10]Ibid., p. 71.
[11]Tony Atkins, "What is Health?" *Health and Development,* summer 1984, p. 5.
[12]Ibid., p. 6.
[13]Nicholas Wolterstorff, "For Justice in Shalom," in *From Christ to the World: Introductory Readings in Christian Ethics*, ed. Wayne G. Boulton, Thomas D. Kennedy and Allen Verhey (Grand Rapids, Mich.: Eerdmans, 1994), p. 251.
[14]Paul Tillich, "The Meaning of Health," in *On Moral Medicine: Theological Perspectives in Medical Ethics*, ed. Stephen E. Lammers and Allen Verhey (Grand Rapids, Mich.: Eerdmans, 1987), p. 162.
[15]Jürgen Moltmann, *The Spirit of Life: A Universal Affirmation* (Minneapolis: Fortress, 1992), p. 191.
[16]Thomas A. Droege, "The Healing Ministry of Jesus as an Example of Wholistic Health Care," in *Theological Roots of Wholistic Health Care*, ed. Granger Westberg (Hinsdale, Ill.: Wholistic Health Centers, 1979), p. 19.
[17]See, for example, J. Birney Dibble, *Outlaw for God: the Story of Esther Bacon* (Hanover, Mass.: Christopher, 1992). An LCA missionary nurse in Liberia, Esther Bacon often taught the missionary doctors how to perform surgery and deliver babies in culturally appropriate ways.
[18]Betty Souther, "Congregational Nurse Practitioner: An Idea Whose Time Has Come," *Journal of Christian Nursing,* winter 1997, pp. 32-34. Souther, the director of the Center for Health Studies at Houston Baptist University, has developed a new Master's of Science

in Nursing program to prepare parish nurses to perform in a role once reserved for physicians.

[19]Florence Nightingale, *Notes on Nursing: What It Is and What It Is Not* (New York: Appleton, 1860), p. 3.

[20]Ruth I. Stoll, *Concepts in Nursing—A Christian Perspective* (Madison, Wis.: Nurses Christian Fellowship, 1990), p. 158.

[21]Karl Barth, "Sickness and Illusion," in *On Moral Medicine: Theological Perspectives in Medical Ethics*, ed. Stephen E. Lammers and Allen Verhey (Grand Rapids, Mich.: Eerdmans, 1987), p. 155.

[22]Daniel Fountain, *Health, the Bible and the Church* (Wheaton, Ill.: Billy Graham Center, 1989), p. 52.

[23]Callahan, "The WHO Definition of 'Health,' " 172.

[24]Halbert L. Dunn, *High Level Wellness* (Arlington, Va.: R. W. Beatty, 1961).

[25]Callahan, "The WHO Definition of 'Health,' " 172.

[26]Stephen E. Lammers and Allen Verhey, eds., *On Moral Medicine: Theological Perspectives in Medical Ethics* (Grand Rapids, Mich.: Eerdmans, 1987), p. 150.

Chapter 11: Hope in Suffering

[1]Stanley Hauerwas, *Naming the Silences: God, Medicine and the Problem of Suffering* (Grand Rapids, Mich.: Eerdmans, 1990), p. 49.

[2]Kenneth Boa, *Cults, World Religions and the Occult* (Wheaton, Ill.: Victor, 1990), pp. 19-20. Also see David Burnett, *The Spirit of Hinduism* (Tunbridge Wells, England: Monarch, 1992), pp. 71-85, 190-204; and George W. Braswell Jr., *Understanding World Religions* (Nashville: Broadman & Holman, 1994), pp. 31-34.

[3]Boa, *Cults, World Religions*, pp. 31-33; see also Braswell, *Understanding World Religions*, pp. 52-58.

[4]Ninan Smart, *Worldviews: Crosscultural Explorations of Human Beliefs* (New York: Scribner's, 1983), pp. 105-7. For nursing implications see "An Asian Patient: How Does Culture Affect Care?" *Journal of Christian Nursing*, summer 1991, pp. 4-9.

[5]John Bowker, *Suffering in the Religions of the World* (Cambridge: Cambridge University Press, 1970), pp. 5-40.

[6]See, for example, Darrell J. Fasching, *Narrative Theology After Auschwitz: From Alienation to Ethics* (Minneapolis: Fortress, 1992).

[7]Bowker, *Suffering*, pp. 99-136.

[8]Boa, *Cults, World Religions*, p. 71; Braswell, *Understanding World Religions*, pp. 111-12.

[9]David Burnett, *Clash of World: A Christian's Handbook on Cultures, World Religions and Evangelism* (Nashville: Thomas Nelson, 1992), pp. 57-68. For nursing implications, see Hsin-chun Mao and Li-ling Yang, "Understanding the Spiritual Needs of Chinese Patients," *Journal of Christian Nursing*, fall 1994, pp. 39-41.

[10]This philosophy found its ultimate expression in the assisted suicide campaign outlined in Derek Humphrey, *Final Exit* (Secaucus, N.Y.: Hemlock Society, 1991); Humphrey, and Jack Kevorkian, *Prescription Medicine: The Goodness of Planned Death* (Buffalo, N.Y.:

Prometheus, 1991).

[11]Barbara Blattner, *Holistic Nursing* (Englewood Cliffs, N. J.: Prentice-Hall, 1981), p. 25.

[12]See, for example, Victoria E. Slater, "Toward an Understanding of Energetic Healing," pt.s 1 and 2 of *Journal of Holistic Nursing*, September 1995, pp. 209-38, and Deirdre Davis Brighman, *Imagery for Getting Well: Clinical Applications of Behavioral Medicine* (San Francisco: Harper & Row, 1984).

[13]Hillstrom, *Testing the Spirits*, p. 193.

[14]Ibid., pp. 164-170.

[15]Mary A. Greenwold Milano and David B. Larson, "The Research Shows: Religion is Healthy," *CMDS Healthwise*, fall 1995, p. 7.

[16]Susan S. and David B. Larson, "Warning: Research Shows Religion Is Good for Your Mental Health," *Christian Counseling Today*, October 1993, p. 28.

[17]David B. Larson and Susan S. Larson, "Clinical Religious Research," *Christian Medical and Dental Society Journal*, summer 1992. Also see Mark Hartwig, "For Good Health, Go to Church," *Focus on the Family Citizen*, June 21, 1993, which has extensive endnotes of research cited.

[18]Rosemary Donley, "Spiritual Dimensions of Health Care: Nursing's Mission," *Nursing and Health Care*, April 1991, pp. 179-80.

[19]Ibid., p. 182.

Chapter 12: The Paradox of Death

[1]Roberta Lyder Paige, letter to Judith Allen Shelly.

[2]Hans Walter Wolff, *Anthropology of the Old Testament* (Philadelphia: Fortress, 1974), 106-7

[3]Stephen H. Travis, *Christian Hope & the Future* (Downers Grove, Ill.: InterVarsity Press, 1980), p. 121.

[4]Larry Richards and Paul Johnson, *Death and the Caring Community: Ministering to the Terminally Ill* (Portland, Ore.: Multnomah, 1980), pp. 61-62.

[5]Ibid., p. 14.

Chapter 13: Nursing as Christian Caring

[1]Roberta Mayhew West, *History of Nursing in Pennsylvania* (Philadelphia: Pennsylvania State Nurses' Association, circa 1932), p. 6.

[2]Emily Hitchens and Lilyan Snow, "Caring: The Moral Response to Suffering," *Christian Scholar's Review*, 1994, p. 309.

[3]Florence Nightingale, *Notes on Nursing: What It Is and What It Is Not* (New York: D. Appleton, 1860), p. 3.

[4]Ibid.

[5]Catherine Herzel, *On Call: Deaconesses Across the World* (New York: Holt, Rinehart, Winston, 1961).

[6]Suzy Farren, *A Call to Care: The Women Who Built Catholic Healthcare in America* (St. Louis, Mo.: Catholic Health Association of the United States, 1996).

[7]C. Golder, *The History of the Deaconess Movement* (Cincinnati: Jennings and Pye, 1903).

[8]"Platform for the ANA," *American Journal of Nursing,* November 1946, p. 729.

[9]"ANA Board Approves a Definition of Nursing Practice," *American Journal of Nursing,* December 1955, p. 1474.

[10]Virginia A. Henderson, *Basic Principles of Nursing Care* (London: International Council of Nurses, 1961), p. 42.

[11]Rozella M. Schlotfeldt, "Defining Nursing: A Historic Controversy," *Nursing Research,* January-February 1987, pp. 64-67.

[12]American Nurses Association, *Nursing: A Social Policy Statement* (Kansas City, Mo.: American Nurses Association, 1980). According to Donna Diers's article "What is Nursing?" in Joanne Comi McCloskey and Helen Kennedy Grace, eds., *Current Issues in Nursing* (St. Louis, Mo.: Mosby, 1997), pp. 6-7, this wording was first adopted by the New York State Nurses Association in 1976, on the recommendation of their counsel that "the diagnostic privilege was the *sine qua non* of independent practice." This statement set off the nursing diagnosis movement with its attempt to establish a unique taxonomy for nursing. The whole process was essentially a political movement to separate nursing from medicine.

[13]American Nurses Association, *Nursing: A Social Policy Statement* (Kansas City, Mo.: American Nurses Association, 1995), p. 6.

[14]Ibid., p. 13.

[15]Ibid., p. 7.

[16]Ibid., p. 12.

[17]"More Power to the Nurses," *Chicago Tribune,* April 14, 1997.

[18]M. Patricia Donahue, *Nursing: The Finest Art,* 2nd ed. (St. Louis: Mosby-Year Book, 1996), pp. 2-7.

[19]Journalist Suzanne Gordon presents some interesting suggestions about this problem of invisibility in "What Nurses Stand For," *Atlantic Monthly,* February 1997, p. 88. "Because nurses observe and cushion what the physician and writer Oliver Sacks has called human beings' falling 'radically into sickness,' they are a reminder of the pain, fear, vulnerability, and loss of control that adults find difficult to tolerate and thus to discuss. . . . [Nurses] are our secret sharers. Even though they are our lifeline during illness, when control is restored the residue of our anxiety and mortality clings to them like dust, and we flee the memory."

[20]Janice M. Morse, Joan Bottorff, Wendy Neander and Shirley Solberg, "Comparative Analysis of Conceptualizations and Theories of Caring," *Image,* summer 1991, pp. 119-26.

[21]Verna Carson, "Caring: The Rediscovery of our Nursing Roots," *Perspectives in Psychiatric Care,* April-June 1994, pp. 4-6.

[22]M. J. Dunlop, "Is a Science of Caring Possible?" *Journal of Advanced Nursing* 11 (1986): 661-70.

[23]Joy A. Bickle, "Starman," *Journal of Christian Nursing,* summer 1995, p. 6.

[24]Roberta Lyder Paige and Jane Finkbiner Looney, "Hospice Care for the Advanced Cancer Patient," *American Journal of Nursing,* November 1977, pp. 1813-15.

Chapter 14: Spiritual Care

[1]Judith Allen Shelly and Sharon Fish, *Spiritual Care: The Nurse's Role* (Downers Grove, Ill.:

InterVarsity Press, 1988), p. 39.

[2]Ruth E Farr, "I'll Just Have to Die," *Journal of Christian Nursing*, fall 1994, pp. 5-6.

[3]*Newsweek*, January 6, 1992, pp. 39-44; *Time*, June 24, 1996, pp. 56-68; *Christianity Today*, January 6, 1997, pp. 20-29. For abstracts on many on the research studies on prayer, see Dale A. Matthews, David B. Larson and Constance P. Barry, *The Faith Factor: An Annotated Bibliography of Clinical Research on Spiritual Subjects* (Arlington, Va.: National Institute for Healthcare Research, 1993).

[4]Larry Dossey, *Prayer is Good Medicine* (San Francisco: HarperSanFrancisco, 1996), p. xiv.

[5]Ibid.

[6]Ibid., p. 31.

[7]Ibid., pp. 180-87.

[8]Based on a Netscape search on March 12, 1997.

[9]Norma Singer, "When Things Go Bump in the Night: A Story of Forgiveness," *Journal of Christian Nursing*, summer 1997, pp. 24-25.

[10]See for example, the winter 1997 issue of the *Journal of Christian Nursing*.

[11]*The Book of Common Prayer* (Greenwich, Conn: Seabury Press, 1928), p. 581.

[12]Irving Hexham, *Concise Dictionary of Religion* (Downers Grove, Ill: InterVarsity Press, 1993), p. 193.

[13]C. O. Buchanan, "Sacrament," in *New Dictionary of Theology*, ed. Sinclair B. Ferguson and David F. Wright (Downers Grove, Ill.: InterVarsity Press, 1988), p. 607.

Chapter 15: Looking to the Future

[1]Judith Allen Shelly, *Health Ministries: A Dual Degree Program for Graduate Nursing Education* (D.Min. diss., Lutheran Theological Seminary, Philadelphia Penn., 1997).

[2]Annette Morrison, "Caring in the Nineties," *Christian Nurse International* 13, no. 1 (1997): 4.

[3]Anne Bishop and John Scudder, "On Being a Neighbor: Nursing's Moral Standard," *Journal of Christian Nursing*, fall 1997, pp. 9-12.

[4]Mary Oesterle and Darlene O'Callaghan, "The Changing Health Care Environment: Impact on Curriculum and Faculty," *N&HC: Perspectives on Community*, March-April 1996, pp. 79-80.

[5]Carol Bence, "The Towel, The Bath," *Journal of Christian Nursing*, fall 1997, p. 24.

Appendix

[1]Adapted and expanded from Arlene Miller, "Evaluating Holistic Health Modalities," in Judith Allen Shelly and Sandra D. John, *Spiritual Dimensions of Mental Health* (Downers Grove, Ill.: InterVarsity Press, 1983), pp. 51-52.

[2]Jean Watson, "A Fulbright in Sweden: Runes, Academics, Archetypal Motifs and Other Things," *Image: Journal of Nursing Scholarship*, spring 1995, p. 72.

[3]Elizabeth Hillstrom, *Testing the Spirits* (Downers Grove, Ill.: InterVarsity Press, 1995), pp. 116-20.

Name Index

Subject Index